MW01235161

*The Skidmore-Roth Outline Series:*

# OBSTETRIC NURSING
## 2nd Edition

*Obstetric Nursing* gives a broad overview of obstetric nursing for nursing students, staff nurses who practice in acute care or prenatal clinic facilities, obstetric nurses, pediatric nurses, and home health . nurses.

An easy-to-read guide to common nursing interventions in obstetric nursing care, *Obstetric Nursing* is divided into four major units: the Prenatal Period, the Intrapartal Period, the Postpartal Period, and the Neonatal Period.

The compact size and outline format helps the user to quickly locate expected signs and symptoms, development changes, adaptations and corresponding assessments, and interventions for the four periods. This format aids the reader to quickly identify necessary nursing actions. In addition, symptoms, consequences, assessments, and interventions for selected prenatal, intrapartal, postpartal and neonatal period complications are presented.

**A SKIDMORE-ROTH PUBLICATION**

Series Editor: Wendy Thompson

Copy Editor: Maura McMillan

Cover design: Veronica Burnett

Typesetting: Affiliated Executive Systems

Notice: The author and the publisher of this volume have taken care to make certain that all information is correct and compatible with the standards generally accepted at the time of publication.

Masten, Yondell

The Skidmore-Roth Outline Series: Obstetric Nursing/Yondell Masten

ISBN 1-56930-070-4

1. Nursing-Handbooks, Manuals

2. Medical-Handbooks, Manuals

SKIDMORE-ROTH PUBLISHING, INC.
2620 S. Parker Road, Suite 147
Aurora, Colorado 80014
1(800) 825-3150

# TABLE OF CONTENTS

## Unit 1

**The Prenatal Period. . . . . . . . . . . . . . . . . 1**

Chapter 1
The Menstrual Cycle and Conception . . . . . . . . 2

Chapter 2
The Signs and Symptoms of Pregnancy . . . . . . . 9

Chapter 3
Physiologic and Developmental Changes
of Pregnancy . . . . . . . . . . . . . . . . . . . . 11

Chapter 4
Maternal and Fetal Assessment . . . . . . . . . . . 21

Chapter 5
Nursing Intervention . . . . . . . . . . . . . . . . 51

Chapter 6
Selected Prenatal Complications . . . . . . . . . . 60

## Unit 2

**The Intrapartal Period . . . . . . . . . . . . . . 79**

Chapter 7
The Process of Birth. . . . . . . . . . . . . . . . 80

Chapter 8
Maternal, Fetal and Neonatal Assessment . . . . . 91

Chapter 9
Nursing Intervention. . . . . . . . . . . . . . . . 101

Chapter 10
Selected Intrapartal Complications . . . . . . . . 105

# Unit 3

**The Postpartal Period** . . . . . . . . . . . . . . **135**

Chapter 11
Physiological and Developmental Changes . . . . 136

Chapter 12
Maternal Assessment . . . . . . . . . . . . . . 143

Chapter 13
Nursing Intervention. . . . . . . . . . . . . . . 151

Chapter 14
Selected Postpartal Complications. . . . . . . . . 157

# Unit 4

**The Neonatal Period** . . . . . . . . . . . . . . . **173**

Chapter 15
Physiological and Developmental
Adaptations . . . . . . . . . . . . . . . . . 174

Chapter 16
Neonatal Assessment . . . . . . . . . . . . . . 185

Chapter 17
Nursing Intervention. . . . . . . . . . . . . . . 194

Chapter 18
Selected Neonatal Complications . . . . . . . . . 200


Appendix A
Summary of Contraceptive Methods . . . . . . . 219

Appendix B
Adolescent Pregnancy and Parenting . . . . . . . 229

Appendix C
Home Care. . . . . . . . . . . . . . . . . . 233

Appendix D
References . . . . . . . . . . . . . . . . . . 236

Index . . . . . . . . . . . . . . . . . . . . 237

# *Unit 1*

## THE PRENATAL PERIOD

*The prenatal period begins with conception and continues to birth. For the purposes of development and assessment, it is divided into three trimesters.*

*The focus of "The Prenatal Period" is the menstrual cycle, conception, embryonic and fetal development, maternal physiological and developmental changes, assessment, prenatal care, and selected common complications of pregnancy.*

CHAPTER 1

# THE MENSTRUAL CYCLE AND CONCEPTION

## THE MENSTRUAL CYCLE

*The term menstrual cycle is really a misnomer. A better term would be the female reproductive cycle (Olds et al, 1996) which consists of cycles of ovulation and menstruation occurring on a continuum. However, since menstrual cycle is the accepted terminology, it will be used with the notation that the process actually includes a hormonal cycle, ovarian cycle, and uterine cycle that overlap and occur at the same time repeatedly from menarche (onset of menstruation or date of first menses) to menopause (cessation of menstruation or date of last menses) roughly every 28 days, unless pregnancy occurs.*

### Hormonal Cycle

1. Gonadotropin-releasing hormone (GnRH) is secreted by the hypothalamus (when estrogen levels are low) and functions to stimulate the anterior pituitary to secrete follicle-stimulating hormone (FSH).

2. FSH (secreted by the anterior pituitary gland) is a gonadotropic hormone that stimulates the ovarian follicle to mature (producing estrogen and maturing the oocyte).

3. Luteinizing hormone (LH) is secreted by the anterior pituitary gland (in response to stimulation by GnRH after the effects of FSH on the follicle have resulted in estrogen production) and causes final maturation of the graafian follicle, ovulation, and formation of luteal tissue (corpus luteum).

4. Estrogen is secreted by the maturing ovarian graafian follicles and
   assists with follicle maturation, expands the uterine blood supply, inhibits FSH production, stimulates LH production, causes the endometrium to proliferate, and increases contraction of the myometrium and fallopian tubes.

5. Progesterone is secreted by the ovarian corpus luteum (formed from the ruptured graafian follicle), reduces the myometrial and fallopian tube contractions caused by estrogen, and prepares the endometrium for implantation by increasing supplies of glycogen, arterial blood, secretory glands, amino acids and water.

**6**. Prostaglandins are produced by the endometrium, play a role in ovulation, and induce progesterone withdrawal and corpus luteum degeneration when pregnancy does not occur.

## Ovarian Cycle

**1. Phase 1:** The follicular phase lasts 14 days in the 28-day cycle but can be shorter or longer in cycles that vary from the "normal" or average 28 days. During this phase, the graafian follicle matures because of the effect of FSH resulting in the growth of the oocyte and production of increasing amounts of estrogen.

Ovulation (rupture of the graafian follicle and extrusion of the mature ovum) occurs 14 days before the next menses (if pregnancy does not occur) in response to the mid-cycle surge of LH. Mittelschmerz (pain at the time of ovulation) may be experienced.

**2. Phase 2:** The luteal phase lasts 14 days regardless of the total length of the cycle and begins following ovulation. The corpus luteum secretes estrogen and progesterone. Degeneration of the corpus luteum begins about one week after ovulation in the absence of pregnancy and menstruation occurs 14 days following ovulation.

## Uterine (or Endometrial) Cycle

**1. Phase 1**: The menstruation phase lasts approximately 1-5 days in the 28-day cycle and results in shedding of the degenerated portion of the endometrium. Estrogen levels are low at this time.

**2. Phase 2**: The proliferative phase occurs during days 6-14 in the 28-day cycle. The endometrium proliferates (endometrium increases in thickness; endometrial glands become larger, longer and more tortuous; blood vessels dilate and become more prominent) under the influence of increasing estrogen production. Cervical secretions become thinner and more alkaline under the influence of increasing estrogen with cervical mucus increasing in elasticity (spinnbarkheit). At the time of ovulation, the cervical mucus exhibits a ferning pattern. Initially, body temperature drops and then rises.

**3. Phase 3:** The secretory phase occurs from days 15-26 in the 28-day cycle. It begins following ovulation. The endometrium becomes secretory, evidenced by marked increase in thickness, increased tissue glycogen, increased dilatation and tortuousness of the glands, secretion of small amounts of endometrial fluid from the glands, and marked increase in uterine vascularity. Progesterone, the dominant hormone produced by the corpus luteum, is responsible for the secretory changes. Body temperature rises slightly following ovulation and remains elevated during the secretory phase.

**4. Phase 4:** The ischemic phase occurs during days 27-28 in the 28-day cycle. If pregnancy has not occurred, the corpus luteum degenerates, resulting in a fall of both estrogen and progesterone secretion, necrosis of portions of the endometrium, rupture of small blood vessels, constriction of spiral arteries, and beginning of menstrual flow.

The relationship of the hormonal, ovarian, and uterine cycles are depicted in **Figure 1**.

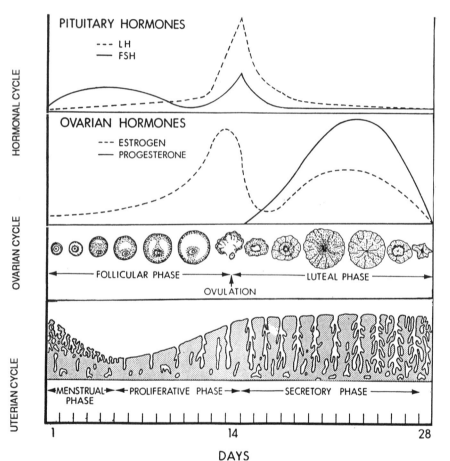

**FIGURE 1:** Menstrual (Reproductive) Cycle. The hormonal, ovarian, and uterine/endometrial cycles are shown as they relate to each other during an average 28-day cycle (Modified, Ortho Pharmaceuticals Education Module, 1974).

# CONCEPTION AND EMBRYONIC/FETAL DEVELOPMENT

## Conception

Conception is the fertilization of the ovum by a spermatozoon. It occurs in the ampulla (outer ⅓ of the fallopian tube). Key events necessary for conception include:

1. Ovulation must occur. The ovum must be mature (first stage of meiosis completed with 23 chromosomes [haploid number] present) and fertile (up to 12-24 hours past ovulation).

2. Spermatozoa must be present. Usually 200-400 million sperm occur in each ejaculation. At least half of the sperm must be motile and greater than 60% must be of normal form. The large number of sperm is required to accomplish the acrosome reaction (deposit of the enzymes hyaluronidase, acrosin, and corona-dispersing enzyme from the head of the sperm to result in perforation of the layer of cells surrounding the ovum). Only one sperm finds a perforation and enters to fertilize the ovum. The one sperm must complete capacitation (removal of the plasma membrane, loss of seminal plasma proteins, and loss of the glycoprotein coat from the head of the sperm) before fertilization can occur. Cervical mucus must be favorable (thin and elastic [Spinnbarkheit of at least 5 cm]) for entrance of sperm into the uterus and movement to the fallopian tubes.

3. Fallopian tubes must be patent and functional (sufficient influence of estrogen to cause development of cilia that are active and peristalsis of tubes for ovum movement. Fimbria must be active to capture the ovum, and tubal mucus must be hospitable).

4. The endometrium must be prepared (by progesterone) for implantation (burrowing into the endometrium until completely covered) of the zygote (fertilized ovum).

## Development

Development of the conceptus includes rapid mitotic cell division (cleavage), development of the membranes and placenta, organogenesis, and continued growth through gestation.

1. The zygote develops into two different types of cells by cleavage during the time from fertilization until implantation is completed. The inner mass of cells will develop into the embryo and amnion (inner membrane) and the outer cells will become the chorion (outer membrane) and the fetal portion of the placenta.

2. The embryo (the conceptus from the beginning of the third week [day 15 since fertilization] through completion of the eighth week) completes organogenesis (formation of all major organ systems).

3. The fetus (the conceptus from the beginning of the ninth week since fertilization until birth) continues development by refining structure and function of the organ systems.

4. The three primary germ layers from which all organ systems develop are the ectoderm (outer layer), mesoderm (intermediate layer), and endoderm (inner layer).

5. The two fetal membranes are the amnion and chorion.

6. The amniotic fluid protects the fetus from injury, helps control the fetus' temperature, and provides freedom of movement to promote musculoskeletal development. The fetus swallows the amniotic fluid, urinates into the fluid, and the fluid flows into and out of the fetal lung. The amount of fluid increases with gestation to approximately 1000 ml at term.

   **Note:** Potential indications of abnormalities exist when the amount of amniotic fluid is too small (oligohydramnios) or excessive (hydramnios).

7. The placenta is developed from the maternal decidua basalis (that portion of the endometrium directly beneath the implanted zygote) and the embryonic/fetal chorionic villi. Placental structure is completely developed by 12 weeks, growth in width is complete at 20 weeks, and growth in thickness occurs until term. The functions of the placenta are the following:

   a. The endocrine function involves production of human chorionic gonadotropin (HCG), human placental lactogen (HPL), progesterone, and the estrogens (estriol is produced primarily by the placenta during pregnancy and estradiol is produced primarily by the ovaries during the menstrual cycle).

      HCG maintains the function of the corpus luteum and promotes increased production of estrogen and progesterone until the placenta can produce sufficient amounts of estrogen and progesterone at about 12 weeks.

      HPL promotes changes in maternal metabolism to make nutrients (protein, glucose, and minerals) available to the embryo and fetus.

      Progesterone helps prepare the endometrium (called *decidua* during pregnancy) for implantation and maintains the endometrium, reduces the contractility of the uterus (caused by estrogens), and stimulates breast alveoli development.

      Estrogen functions proliferatively in pregnancy also. It is responsible for stimulating uterine and breast enlargement, causing proliferation of breast glandular tissue, increasing blood supply to the uterus and placenta, and causing uterine contractility.

    **b.** The metabolic function includes respiration, nourishment, excretion, and storage of nutrients and minerals for fetal use.

**8.** Fetal system development proceeds throughout the fetal gestational period to result in refined and functional systems at birth.

    **a.** The fetal circulatory system functions to supply oxygen and nutrients and to remove waste products. The placenta provides oxygenated blood to the fetus through the umbilical vein in the umbilical cord. Deoxygenated blood returns from the fetus through the two umbilical arteries. Since the fetal lungs do not function to oxygenate fetal blood and the fetal liver does not function for detoxification, three circulatory bypasses are present in the fetus to shunt most of the blood (except a small amount needed for nourishment of the lungs and liver) past the lungs and liver. The three bypasses are:

    The foramen ovale shunts most of the blood entering the right atrium into the left atrium where it then enters the left ventricle and is pumped into the aorta.

    The ductus arteriosus shunts most of the blood entering the pulmonary artery (from the right ventricle) into the aorta.

    The ductus venosus shunts most of the blood from the umbilical vein past the liver and into the inferior vena cava.

    **b.** The respiratory system needs almost the entire fetal period to complete development of adequate numbers of alveoli that are mature enough to produce sufficient amounts of surfactant (wetting agent) and to permit adequate gas exchange. Fetal lung movements move amniotic fluid in and out of the lungs during fetal life.

    **c.** The fetal renal system begins functioning during fetal life and produces urine which is present in amniotic fluid. However, the kidneys still are not able to concentrate urine at term and the glomerular filtration rate is still low.

    **d.** The fetal neurological system develops rapidly during the prenatal period and continues development for two years after birth. The fetus responds to sounds and firm touch in utero.

    **e.** The fetal gastrointestinal system is mature enough to produce enough digestive enzymes for digestion to occur about a month before term.

    **f.** The fetal liver does not function during fetal life, but it does develop stores of glycogen and iron for extrauterine life.

**g.** The fetal endocrine system begins functioning during fetal life and produces increasing amounts of hormones throughout gestation. The fetus produces its own thyroxine, adrenal hormones, and insulin early in gestation.

**h.** The fetal musculoskeletal system development permits movement early in gestation even though maternal perception of fetal movements does not occur until approximately the 20th week.

**i.** The fetal integumentary system continues development throughout the fetal period. Vernix caseosa (cheesy, protective substance) covers the fetus by clinging to the lanugo (fine, downy hair) from about 24 weeks until near term.

**j.** The fetal immune system begins production of albumin and globulin during the third trimester and can fight infection at birth but remains relatively immature even at term.

## Teratogens

Teratogens are any chemical, agent, or organism that cause an adverse effect on the development of the embryo or fetus. Examples of chemicals that impact the conceptus adversely include drugs (e.g., "street" drugs, Accutane, androgens, warfarin, dicumarol, antithyroid drugs, chemotherapy drugs, diethylstilbestrol, Lithium, phenytoin, Streptomycin, Tetracycline, Thalidomide, valproic acid), alcohol, and cigarette smoke. Agents that adversely affect development include radiation, lead, and organic mercury. Organisms include cytomegalovirus, rubella, syphilis, toxoplasmosis, and varicella. In addition, exposure to maternal diseases such as diabetes mellitus and phenylketonuria adversely impact development.

During the zygote period of development, the outcome of teratogenic exposure tends to be "all-or-none" (death if all cells are affected or no lasting effect if not all cells are affected) because all of the cells are alike during that period of development. During organogenesis (embryonic period), the adverse impact is structural and the adverse outcome tends to be evident in the organ system that was undergoing rapid differentiation at the time of exposure. Exposure during the fetal period of development tends to impact organ system function.

CHAPTER 2

# THE SIGNS AND SYMPTOMS OF PREGNANCY

*The signs and symptoms of pregnancy as they relate to the diagnosis of pregnancy can be classified as presumptive, probable, and positive. Presumptive symptoms are subjective symptoms noticed and reported by the pregnant woman. Probable symptoms are objective symptoms noticed by the health provider, but they may be due to causes other than pregnancy. Positive symptoms are objective symptoms that can be caused only by the fetus.*

## PRESUMPTIVE SYMPTOMS

Presumptive symptoms reported by the woman include amenorrhea (missed menstrual period), nausea and/or vomiting ("morning sickness"), urinary frequency (especially nocturia), breast tenderness and/or sensitivity, quickening (maternal perception of first fetal movements), and fatigue. The presumptive symptoms may be caused by endocrine disorders, gastrointestinal disorders, infections, flatus, or life-style changes. Thus, they are considered suspicious of pregnancy rather than diagnostic of pregnancy.

## PROBABLE SYMPTOMS

Probable symptoms observed by the health provider include changes in skin, positive pregnancy tests, and changes in the uterus, cervix, and vagina. Skin changes include facial chloasma ("mask of pregnancy" pigmentation), a linea nigra (pigmentation of the line dividing the abdomen into left and right halves), and breast, buttock, and/or abdominal striae ("stretch marks").

Pregnancy tests use the first voided morning urine specimen (because it is most concentrated) or serum to identify the presence of HCG indicating pregnancy. Because false positive results can occur, or false negative results if the pregnancy is so recent that the HCG levels are not detected, the pregnancy tests are not considered positive diagnosis of pregnancy at this time.

Uterine, cervical, and vaginal changes suggestive of pregnancy include the following:

1. **Chadwick's sign** is the bluish hue of the cervix and vagina caused by increased vasocongestion of the pelvic vessels supplying the uterus. Some professionals consider Chadwick's sign a presumptive rather than a probable symptom of pregnancy.

2. **Goodell's sign** is softening of the cervix noted on pelvic exam by the health provider.

3. **Hegar's sign** is softening of the isthmus of the uterus noted on bimanual exam.

4. **McDonald's sign** is ability of health provider to easily flex the cervix and uterine body against each other.

5. **Change in uterine shape** from the usual pear-shape to a more globular shape is noted by the health provider on pelvic exam.

6. **Palpation of Braxton-Hicks contractions** by the health provider occurs after the end of the first trimester.

7. **Ballottement** is rebound tapping by the fetus on the cervix or lower uterine segment palpated by the examiner. Ballottement is elicited by the examiner tapping the cervix with two fingers intra-vaginally. The fetus responds to the tapping by moving to the uterine fundus and then returning to tap on the cervix.

8. **Palpation of the fetal outline** by the health provider is possible during the second half of pregnancy.

An additional probable symptom is progressive abdominal enlargement observed by the health provider. Because probable symptoms can be caused by tumors, oral contraceptives, obesity, and conditions causing increased vascular congestion they are not considered diagnostic of pregnancy.

# POSITIVE SYMPTOMS

Positive symptoms include auscultation of the fetal heartbeat by fetoscope or doptone, palpation of fetal movement by the health provider, and demonstration of the fetal outline by ultrasound (or x-rays). Since these objective symptoms are caused only by the fetus, they are considered positive or diagnostic symptoms. Auscultation of the fetal heart rate with the doptone is usually possible at 10-12 weeks unless the mother is obese. The fetal heartbeat can be seen by ultrasound at about seven to eight weeks. Auscultation of the fetal heart rate by fetoscope is possible at 20 weeks.

## CHAPTER 3
# PHYSIOLOGIC AND DEVELOPMENTAL CHANGES OF PREGNANCY

## PHYSIOLOGIC CHANGES OF PREGNANCY

*Physiologic changes of pregnancy affect every maternal organ and system in order to support growth of the embryo/fetus. The changes are stimulated by hormonal and uterine/fetal growth influences.*

**Reproductive system changes** involve the uterus, cervix, vagina, ovaries, and breasts. Changes for each structure are summarized below.

1. **The Uterus**

   **Uterine enlargement** stimulated by increasing amounts of estrogen and progesterone occurs primarily by hypertrophy and to a much smaller extent by hyperplasia. **Hypertrophy** is increase in cell size. **Hyperplasia** is increase in cell number. The uterus increases in size from an approximately fist-sized (or small pear-sized) pelvic organ to a large abdominal organ capable of containing a term fetus and about 1000 ml of amniotic fluid.

   **Uterine shape** changes from that of a small inverted pear at the time of conception, to the shape of a sphere in the second trimester, and finally to a large oval shape in the third trimester.

   **Uterine consistency** changes throughout pregnancy. At the time of conception, the uterus is firm (almost a solid organ) with a uterine wall that is about ½ inch (or 13 mm) thick and remains rather thick during early pregnancy. By term, the uterus is soft with the uterine wall thinning to about 5 mm, thus, facilitating palpation of the fetus.

   **Uterine position** changes from being completely contained in the pelvis to being an abdominal organ during the second and third trimesters.

   **Uterine tone** changes from firm at the beginning of pregnancy to soft as the uterine wall thins. In addition, uterine tone changes from soft to firm when uterine contractions occur. Contractions can be either **Braxton-Hicks** or true labor contractions.

2. **The Cervix**

   Cervical changes are stimulated by estrogen and include hypertrophy, hyperplasia, and increase in glandular tissue activity. The cervical glands increase in number and secrete an increased amount of thick mucus which forms the mucous plug. The mucous plug provides protection against ascending bacteria and other organisms. The cervix develops a bluish hue and becomes soft early in pregnancy. It may also become friable (bleed easily when touched).

3. **The Vagina**

   Vaginal changes involve hypertrophy, hyperplasia, and increased vascularization changes that are stimulated by the influence of estrogen. The overall effect of the changes causes the vaginal mucosa to increase in thickness, increase the amount of vaginal secretions, and develop a bluish hue (**Chadwick's sign** of pregnancy). The increase in secretions helps prevent vaginal infections by making the pH more acidic.

4. **The Ovaries**

   Ovarian changes include continued growth of the corpus luteum and continued production of estrogen and progesterone until about the 12th week of gestation. By 12 weeks the placenta is capable of taking over the production of estrogen and progesterone from the corpus luteum. Then, the corpus luteum regresses in a manner similar to that of the menstrual cycle in the latter part of the luteal phase. During pregnancy, the cyclic maturation of follicles and ovulation cease because of the high levels of estrogen.

5. **The Breasts**

   Breast changes include hypertrophy, hyperplasia, and increased vascularity changes that prepare the breast for lactation at the end of pregnancy. Evidence of the changes includes increase in breast size, increase in tissue nodularity, increase in nipple and areola pigmentation, increase in size of Montgomery's glands, possible development of striae, and in the first trimester, increased tenderness and sensitivity of the breasts.

   **Cardiovascular system changes** include blood volume, cardiac output, blood pressure, and coagulation changes. The changes result from hormonal and mechanical stimulation.

   1. **Blood volume changes** include a progressive increase in volume during pregnancy resulting in an increase of almost 50% by about 32 weeks gestation. Both plasma and blood cell components contribute to this increase. The more rapid increase in plasma than red blood cells can result in pseudoanemia or **physiologic anemia of pregnancy.** White blood cell (WBC)

production increases slightly during pregnancy resulting in elevated WBC values for pregnancy, especially during the third trimester and labor.

2. **Cardiac output changes** result from the increase in blood volume. The amount of increase is 30%-50% with the peak increase occurring by 28-30 weeks. Increased flow occurs to the reproductive system, the GI system, the renal system, and the integumentary system. In addition, the pulse gradually increases by 10-15 beats per minute by 20 weeks.

3. **Blood pressure changes** vary among individuals. In general, the blood pressure during the first trimester is approximately the same as during the nonpregnant state. Because of the increase in vasodilation in the second trimester, the blood pressure decreases slightly. Then, in the third trimester, the blood pressure values return to values similar to those of the first trimester. In addition, during the second half of pregnancy, the uterus is heavy enough to reduce flow through the inferior vena cava when the expectant mother is supine. The compression of the inferior vena cava between the gravid uterus and maternal spine is called **vena cava syndrome or supine hypotension syndrome** and results in signs and symptoms of hypotension in the mother and fetus.

4. **Coagulation changes** include a decrease in fibrinolytic activity, an increase in fibrin, and an increase in clotting factors. These changes result in an increase in clotting capability during pregnancy. However, clotting time remains approximately the same as in non-pregnancy. The increase in clotting tendency is protective.

**Respiratory system changes** involve mechanical, functional, and basal metabolism changes. These changes are stimulated by the hormones estrogen and progesterone and by structural changes necessitated by the enlarging uterus.

1. **Mechanical changes** include an elevation in the diaphragm and an increase in the transverse diameter of the thorax. These changes contribute to the change to thoracic rather than abdominal breathing.

2. **Functional changes** include a decreased threshold for carbon dioxide, an increased tidal volume, an increased respiratory minute volume, and only a slightly increased respiratory rate. These changes result in the **hyperventilation of pregnancy** that maintains a decrease in the concentration of carbon dioxide at the alveolar level and the perception of shortness of breath by the expectant mother. Even though there is no decrease in respiratory function during pregnancy, the expectant mother is at greater risk for respiratory diseases than she is when she is not

pregnant. In addition, estrogen results in an increase in vascularity of the nose and can cause nasal stuffiness, nosebleeds, and voice changes.

3. **Basal metabolism changes** result in an increase in the basal metabolism rate (BMR). The increased BMR meets the increased oxygen needs of the fetus and maternal cardiac workload.

**Gastrointestinal system changes** involve appetite changes, nausea and vomiting, mouth and gum changes, decreased peristalsis, decreased motility, acid production changes, and hepatic changes. The changes are caused by hormones and pressure of the growing uterus.

1. **Appetite changes** may include a decrease in appetite during episodes of nausea and vomiting. Then after "morning sickness" resolves, there is an increase in appetite, especially after the first trimester.

2. **Nausea and vomiting changes** of early pregnancy vary among individual women. It is usually precipitated by a decrease in blood glucose level because of use of glucose for embryonic and fetal development and may occur because of fatigue. HCG is also thought to play a role in the nausea and vomiting of early pregnancy, especially since both the nausea and vomiting and HCG levels decrease at about three months gestation.

3. **Mouth and gum changes** include increased vascularity and edema due to the effects of estrogen. For some women the gums may bleed easily and some women may notice an increase in saliva. If the mother does not practice dental hygiene, she is at risk for gingivitis.

4. **Peristalsis and motility changes** include decreased smooth muscle tone, decreased smooth muscle motility, decreased and/or reverse peristalsis, relaxation of the cardioesophageal sphincter, displacement of the stomach, and increased stomach emptying time. These effects are primarily due to the effect of progesterone on smooth muscle and a contribution by the impact of the pressure of the enlarging uterus as pregnancy progresses. The mother may experience "heartburn," flatulence, constipation, and possible development of hemorrhoids as a consequence of these changes.

5. **Acid production changes** include an increase in acidity of gastric contents due to an increase in gastrin production by the placenta. Gastrin is a hormone which causes the increase in pepsin and hydrochloric acid secretion under certain conditions.

6. **Hepatic changes** include decreased gallbladder muscle tone, increased emptying time of the gallbladder, and a slight hyper-cholesterolemia caused by the smooth muscle relaxation effects

of progesterone. As a consequence, the mother may develop gallstones.

**Renal system changes** involve structural changes, functional changes, and fluid and electrolyte changes. Hormonal influences and pressure from the enlarging uterus contribute to the changes.

1. **Structural changes** may include dilatation of each renal pelvis and ureter, and changes in bladder capacity and sensitivity. The consequence of renal pelvis and ureter dilatation is urine stasis which may increase the risk for urinary tract infection. The pressure of the enlarging uterus on the bladder (especially in the first trimester and in the latter part of the third trimester with fetal presenting part engagement) results in nocturia, increased frequency and increased urgency.

2. **Functional changes** include increased renal plasma flow and glomerular filtration rate (GFR), a decrease in blood urea nitrogen (BUN) and plasma creatinine levels, and decreased renal threshold for glucose. The decrease in BUN and plasma creatinine occur because the increase in GFR increases the clearance of urea and creatinine. Also, glucose is rapidly filtered out of the urine because of the increased GFR and renal plasma flow, but glucose is not reabsorbed as rapidly and may appear in the urine without indicating the occurrence of hyperglycemia. Renal function is improved in the side-lying position, especially the left side-lying position because of increased renal perfusion. Renal function is adversely affected by the supine position because renal perfusion is decreased by supine hypotension (or **vena cava syndrome**).

3. **Fluid and electrolyte changes** include changes to maintain sodium and water balance. Aldosterone secretion by the adrenal glands increases early in pregnancy. Aldosterone facilitates reabsorption of sodium. Excretion of water is more efficient in early pregnancy than later in pregnancy. Water retention can result in edema. The extra water is used to increase maternal blood volume and to transport nutrients to the fetus. Excessive fluid retention may occur later in pregnancy and is considered undesirable when it is accompanied by the presence of enough protein in the urine to indicate a disease process and by blood pressure elevation.

**Integumentary system changes** involve pigmentation, striae, hair and nail growth, and sweat gland and sebaceous gland activity as the most common changes. The changes are due to hormonal and mechanical stimulation.

1. **Pigmentation changes** include increased pigmentation of the areola of the breast, development of **chloasma (mask of pregnancy)**, and appearance of the **linea nigra.** Melanocyte stimulating hormone causes the increased pigmentation.

2. **Striae changes** (stretch marks) appear because of mechanical stretching separation of the collagen tissue beneath the skin. Striae occur on the abdomen, thigh, and/or breast.

3. **Hair and nail growth** changes may result in increased length of nails and increased thickness of hair. Estrogen is thought to be the cause of the change in hair and nail growth.

4. **Sweat gland and sebaceous gland changes** include an increase in activity during pregnancy. The consequences may be an increase in body odor, increase in oily skin, and/or development of acne in some women.

**Metabolic system changes** involve nitrogen, fats, carbohydrates, iron, and calcium. Metabolic changes are mediated by hormones.

1. **Nitrogen changes** include the increase in storage of nitrogen throughout pregnancy. Nitrogen is supplied by proteins and is utilized in early pregnancy for maternal tissue growth (hyperplasia and hypertrophy) and for fetal growth in the second half of pregnancy.

2. **Fats** are absorbed more efficiently during pregnancy. They are utilized for maternal energy, fetal deposits (especially late in pregnancy), and preparation for lactation.

3. **Carbohydrates** are utilized for embryonic and fetal growth, energy, sparing protein, and preventing ketosis. Demand for carbohydrates, especially complex carbohydrates, increases during the second and third trimesters.

4. **Iron** is utilized to prevent anemia, increased RBC production, and for fetal storage (especially during the third trimester).

5. **Calcium** is stored throughout pregnancy. It is utilized for fetal teeth and bone calcification.

**Musculoskeletal system changes** involve collagen and connective tissue changes, muscle tone changes, and a shift in center of gravity. The changes occur because of hormonal influences and progressive increase in size of the growing uterus.

1. **Collagen and connective tissue changes** include softening of the tissues. The result is a widening of the symphysis pubis and relaxation of the joints of the pelvis. The change is thought to be caused by relaxin and possibly progesterone. The purpose is to

increase the pelvic diameters to facilitate passage of the fetus at birth. The effect on the mother is a progressive waddling-type gait due to mobility of the pelvis, especially near term.

2. **Muscle tone changes** include some decrease in tone. The decrease in tone of the abdominal recti muscles and the pressure of the enlarging uterus can result in **diastasis recti abdominis** (a separation of the rectus muscles).

3. **The shift in center of gravity** is caused by the progressive growth of the uterus and weight of the uterine contents. The increased weight protruding further and further in front of the mother causes a progressive shift in her center of gravity. The consequence is an increased tendency to fall or a loss of balance, especially with sudden position change.

**Neurologic system changes** that occur in pregnancy in some women include carpal tunnel syndrome, acroesthesia, backache, faintness, and muscle cramps. The cause of such changes is not always well understood and may be due to pressure on or strain of a nerve plexus or due to edema.

1. **Carpal tunnel syndrome** is pain, burning, or tingling of the palm that may extend to the elbow. It is thought to be due to edema that compresses the median nerve as it passes through the carpal tunnel.

2. **Acroesthesia** is a numbness and tingling of the hands due to a stooped shoulder posture that places traction on the brachial nerve plexus.

3. **Backache** because of lordosis in an effort to compensate for the shift in center of gravity may result in back pain caused by traction or pressure on nerve roots.

4. **Faintness**, especially in early pregnancy, may be caused by hypoglycemia, postural hypotension, or vasomotor instability.

5. **Muscle cramps** due to hypocalcemia are the result of muscle tetany.

**Endocrine system changes** involve thyroid, parathyroid, pancreas, pituitary, adrenal, and hormonal changes.

1. **Thyroid changes** include an increase in thyroid gland hormone production and activity. The increase in activity is caused by hyperplasia and increased vascularity. Oxygen consumption and increased BMR occur in response to increased metabolic activity associated with the pregnancy.

2. **Parathyroid changes** include increase in parathyroid size and hormone production. Increase in hormone production is required for calcium metabolism involved in fetal skeleton development.

3. **Pancreas changes** include increased production of insulin as pregnancy progresses. Estrogen, progesterone, cortisol, and human placental lactogen (human chorionic somatomammotropin) decrease the ability of the maternal tissues to use insulin. This consequence is thought to be protective in that it assures the availability of glucose for fetal use. As a consequence, the pancreas must produce progressively more insulin as the pregnancy progresses to compensate for the effects of the increase in production of estrogen, progesterone, cortisol, and HPL. If the pancreas cannot produce enough insulin, maternal diabetes mellitus occurs during pregnancy.

4. **Pituitary changes** include cessation of FSH and LH production and increased production of prolactin, and late in pregnancy, oxytocin. Prolactin may contribute to breast development during pregnancy and stimulates milk production after birth. It does not cause milk production during pregnancy because of the high levels of estrogen. Oxytocin production during labor increases the intensity of uterine contractions and postpartally stimulates let down (contraction of the smooth muscle of the lactiferous ducts of the breast to move milk to the lactiferous sinuses).

5. **Adrenal changes** include increased circulating levels of cortisol and aldosterone. Cortisol influences metabolism of carbohydrates and proteins. Aldosterone helps maintain fluid balance by regulating reabsorption of sodium by the kidney.

6. **Hormonal changes** that are related to the condition of being pregnant include production of human chorionic gonadotropin (HCG), human placental lactogen (HPL), estrogen, progesterone, relaxin, and prostaglandin.

   a. **HCG** is secreted by chorionic villi during early pregnancy and stimulates continued hormone production by the corpus luteum to prevent regression of the uterine endometrium.

   b. **HPL** is an insulin antagonist and also facilitates availability of glucose for embryonic/fetal growth and use of fat for maternal energy needs.

   c. **Estrogen** stimulates reproductive system hypertrophy, breast ductal development, and increased vascularity to reproductive organs.

   d. **Progesterone** acts as an antagonist to the estrogen induced contractility of the uterus, causes smooth muscle relaxation, and prepares the breast for lactation by stimulating breast glandular tissue development.

Estrogen and progesterone work either synergistically (estrogen begins the change and progesterone completes the change) or antagonistically (progesterone reduces the effect of estrogen to achieve a balance).

e. **Relaxin** is primarily responsible for promoting relaxation of pelvic joints and softening of the symphysis pubis to facilitate passage of the fetus through the pelvis during birth.

f. **Prostaglandin** function in pregnancy is not well defined. It is known that prostaglandin does cause uterine contractions and effacement of the cervix. It may be responsible for initiating labor.

# DEVELOPMENTAL CHANGES OF PREGNANCY

Developmental changes of pregnancy include the emotional and psychological changes that occur because of pregnancy. Developmental changes are influenced by the mother's partner, family, culture, life experiences, and society. There are specific developmental tasks to be completed during the pregnancy.

**Influences** that impact the developmental changes of pregnancy vary and may be positive or negative. If the expectant mother can depend on her partner to support her through the pregnancy, through the birthing process, and in caring for the infant/child, the impact is usually positive. However, if the partner is not pleased about the pregnancy or abandons the mother and infant, the influence is negative.

**Family influences** impact the mother's view of the pregnancy because of the manner in which pregnancies were welcomed or resented by the family as the mother was growing up. If each pregnancy and child were desired, the mother will probably view her pregnancy as a positive experience. However, if her mother identified each pregnancy as an additional burden, the expectant mother may view her pregnancy as a problem or burden.

**Cultural influences** include beliefs, roles, activities, and behavior that are appropriate for pregnancy. Numerous "old wives tales" about pregnancy originate in cultural influences.

**Life experiences** of the mother influence the pregnancy. If the mother has felt capable of coping with experiences in the past, she will most likely feel capable of coping with the pregnancy and enter into preparation for birthing and parenting. However, if the mother has felt incapable of coping with past life experiences, she may perceive that she will have difficulty coping with the pregnancy and birthing experience.

**Social influences** impact the pregnancy in that expectant mothers tend to adopt the perception of pregnancy that was current during their youth and during the current pregnancy. Examples include the past view that pregnancy is confining and that pregnant women should not be involved in social events. Another example would be the current view that expectant mothers and their support persons should attend childbirth preparation classes.

**The tasks of pregnancy** occur throughout the period of pregnancy and promote preparation of the expectant family to parent the infant and child. There are three primary tasks of pregnancy, acceptance of the pregnancy, acceptance of the baby, and acceptance of motherhood. The tasks can be roughly categorized according to the trimesters of pregnancy.

1. **Acceptance of the pregnancy** is usually completed by the end of the first trimester. Initially the mother is usually ambivalent about the pregnancy even though she may have been trying to become pregnant. Evidence that the mother has accepted the pregnancy includes her verbalization to others that she is pregnant and her wearing of maternity clothes.

2. **Acceptance of the baby** is usually completed in the second trimester. The mother begins viewing the fetus as a baby rather than a pregnancy. She becomes excited about having a baby, develops a vision of her fantasy child, and begins purchasing things for the baby. She changes her diet and activities "for the baby."

3. **Acceptance of motherhood** occurs by the end of the third trimester. The mother indicates readiness to be a mother and she views the baby as a separate individual from herself. She makes the final preparations for the arrival of the baby and prepares for birth and motherhood.

Common emotional changes of pregnancy include ambivalence at the time of confirmation of the pregnancy, introversion, and mood swings.

1. The initial emotion for the majority of expectant mothers is **ambivalence**. The duration of the ambivalence seems to depend on the amount of change that having a baby will necessitate in her life.

2. **Introversion** is commonly experienced by expectant mothers. The focus inward on herself and on her body progresses through pregnancy and peaks during labor. As she becomes more introverted, the mother appears to be more sensitive and to have more difficulty making decisions.

3. **Mood swings** are a commonly recognized emotional response of expectant mothers to pregnancy. The mothers experience extreme joyful feelings one minute and begin crying the next minute without being able to give a reason for the tears. Hormonal changes are thought to be partially responsible for the mood swings.

# CHAPTER 4
# MATERNAL AND FETAL ASSESSMENT

*Prenatal care promotes improved maternal and fetal outcomes of pregnancy because it focuses on early identification of alterations in the health of the mother and fetus, treatment of alterations in health, promoting positive health habits (including nutrition), and recommendations for birthing preparation. The expectant mother makes scheduled prenatal visits to her health provider. The usual schedule for "normal" pregnancy is once each month from diagnosis to 32 weeks gestation, every other week from 32 weeks to 36 weeks and once each week from 36 weeks until birth. If alterations in health occur or if the expectant mother is classified as "high risk," prenatal visits will be scheduled more often.*

## MATERNAL ASSESSMENT

Maternal assessment includes an initial maternal history and physical examination, episodic histories and well-being assessments through-out the pregnancy, and initial plus progressive risk assessments. The pregnancy history involves the use of several new terms. Definitions of the terms are as follows:

1. **Abortion** is the passage of the products of conception prior to completion of 20 weeks of pregnancy. It may be spontaneous (termed "miscarriage" by the general public) or induced (a "termination").

2. **Antenatal or antepartum** is the period from conception to the onset of labor.

3. **Gestation** is the condition of being pregnant and usually refers to the number of weeks of pregnancy based on the first day of the last normal menstrual period or on ultrasound dating of the pregnancy.

4. **Gravida** is the number of times the mother has been pregnant.

5. **Intrapartum** is the period of time from the onset of labor until the birth of the baby and delivery of the placenta.

6. **Multigravida** is a woman who is pregnant for at least the second time or has been pregnant two or more times.

7. **Neonate** is an infant that is between birth and 28 days of age.

8. **Neonatal period** is the time from the birth of the infant until 28 days of life.

9. **Multipara** is a woman who has experienced two or more pregnancies resulting in vaginal or cesarean section births which were more than 20 weeks gestation.

10. **Nulligravida** is a woman who has had zero pregnancies (never been pregnant).

11. **Nullipara** is a woman who has experienced zero pregnancies resulting in a birth of more than 20 weeks gestation.

12. **Para** is the number of pregnancies a woman has experienced which resulted in births of more than 20 weeks gestation.

13. **Postpartum** is the period from birth to 42 days (6 weeks) after birth.

14. **Prenatal period** is the time from conception to birth.

15. **Primigravida** is a woman who is pregnant for the first time.

16. **Primipara** is a woman who has experienced one vaginal or cesarean birth which was more than 20 weeks gestation.

17. **Stillbirth** is the birth of a dead fetus that was more than 20 weeks gestation.

## History

The **initial maternal history** must be thorough to identify factors that could cause or contribute to alterations in maternal/fetal well-being or adverse outcomes. Components of the initial history include:

- Past medical history
- Current medical history and review of systems
- Sexual history
- Gynecologic history
- Obstetric history
- Occupational history
- Family medical history
- Social and cultural history
- Developmental history
- Partner's past medical history
- Partner's current medical history
- Partner's sexual history
- Partner's occupational history
- Partner's family medical history

## Risk Factors

**Risk factors** are obtained from the initial and episodic histories. The risk factors can be divided into personal, life-style, health, and past history factors and include:

## Maternal Personal Factors:

- Low socioeconomic status
- Low educational level
- High parity (> 4)
- Age < 16 or > 35 years
- Nullipara 35 or > 35 years of age
- Multipara 40 or > 40 years of age
- Pregnancy within 3 months of previous birth
- Pre-pregnant weight < 100 lbs. or > 200 lbs.
- Short stature (< 5 feet)

## Maternal Life-Style Factors:

- Inadequate nutrition
- Smoking
- Alcohol use
- Addicting drug use

## Maternal Health Factors:

- Anemia
- Multiple gestation
- Hemorrhage in present pregnancy
- Preterm rupture of membranes
- Sickle cell disease or trait
- Diabetes mellitus or gestational diabetes
- Cardiac disease
- Kidney disease
- Hypertension
- Thyroid disease

- TORCH infections (toxoplasmosis, rubella, CMV, Herpes Type II)
- Syphilis, gonorrhea, chlamydia
- Tuberculosis
- Tumors (malignant or premalignant)
- Epilepsy
- Mental retardation
- Psychiatric disorder

## Maternal Past History Factors:

- Cephalopelvic Disproportion (CPD)
- Cesarean birth
- Prolonged labor
- Reproductive track anomaly (incompetent cervix, cervical or uterine malformation, tubal occlusion or malformation, ovarian mass, endometriosis)
- Diabetes mellitus (including gestational diabetes)
- Anemia
- Hemorrhage
- Bleeding or clotting disorder
- Drug or alcohol abuse
- Pregnancy-induced hypertension (PIH)
- Preterm birth (2 or more)
- Abortion (2 or more consecutive spontaneous)
- Term stillbirth (2 or more)
- Previous Infant with:
  - Rh or ABO incompatibility
  - Birth defect(s)
  - Mental retardation
  - Metabolic disorder
  - Macrosomia (at least 9 lb or 4032 g)

## Maternal Initial Physical Assessment

A thorough initial physical assessment provides baseline data for comparison of changes during pregnancy and identification of alterations in well-being during subsequent scheduled assessments. In general the initial assessment involves general physical assessment activities plus a specific pregnancy assessment. Components of the initial maternal physical assessment include:

- Vital signs
- Weight
- Height
- Head and scalp
- Eyes
- Ears
- Nose
- Sinuses
- Mouth, teeth, throat
- Neck and thyroid gland
- Lymph nodes
- Chest, heart and lungs
- Spine and costovertebral angle (CVA) tenderness
- Breasts
- Abdomen, fetal heart rate, and fundal height (if applicable)
- Skin, extremities, Homan's sign
- Pelvic, anus, and rectum

At the initial physical assessment visit, several laboratory assessments are made. The initial laboratory studies include:

- CBC
- Syphilis test
- Rubella screen
- Hepatitis B surface antigen screen
- Blood type and Rh
- Rh antibody screen (Rh negative mother)
- HIV screen
- Sickle cell screen (black mother)

- Urinalysis (including microscopic exam) and culture
- Gonorrhea and chlamydia culture
- Pap smear

The **Estimated Date of Delivery (EDD)** is determined at the initial visit. It is determined using Nägele's Rule and compared with the uterine size as evaluated by the pelvic examination. Nägele's Rule uses the first day of the last menstrual period (LMP) or the first day of the last normal menstrual period (LNMP), if the last menstrual period was abnormal in terms of amount or duration of menses. The EDD determined by Nägele's Rule adds 7 days to the first day of the LMP, subtracts 3 months from the month of the LMP and adds 1 year to the year of the LMP. The calculated EDD is then considered correct within 2 weeks. An example would be a client with the first day of her LMP being July 4, 1997. The calculation would be the following:

| Month | Day |
|-------|-----|
| LMP  7 | 4 |
| EDD -3 | +7 |
| 4 | 11 |

Thus, the EDD would be April 11, 1998, and birth could be expected within 2 weeks before or 2 weeks after April 11. If the uterine size is approximately the same as the calculated weeks of gestation, then the data indicate uterine size and EDD date consistency (abbreviated as size-date consistency or S=D).

## Episodic History and Well-Being Assessment

Episodic history and well-being assessments are made at each subsequent prenatal visit. The episodic history includes a summary of physical and emotional problems and complaints since the previous prenatal visit. Specific questions can be asked based on expected needs of each trimester. The following is a sample list by trimester:

**First Trimester:**
1. Discomforts
   - Breast changes
   - Family dynamics
   - Fatigue
   - Gingivitis
   - Leukorrhea
   - Nasal stuffiness and/or epistaxis
   - Nausea and/or vomiting
   - Psychosocial responses

**2**. Self Care
- Exercise

- Nutrition

- Rest and relaxation

**3**. Warning or Danger Signs
- Bleeding

- Burning on urination

- Chills and fever

- Cramping

- Diarrhea

- Persistent, severe vomiting

**Second Trimester:**
**1.** Discomforts
- Faintness

- Family dynamics

- Gastrointestinal distress

- Gingivitis

- Neuromuscular distress

- Palpitations

- Psychosocial responses

- Skeletal distress

- Skin changes

- Varicosities

**2.** Self Care
- Exercise

- Nutrition

- Rest and relaxation

- Sexuality

**3.** Warning or Danger Signs
- Bleeding

- Burning on urination

- Chills and fever

- Decreased or absent fetal movements

- Diarrhea

- Persistent, severe vomiting

– Ruptured membranes

**Third Trimester**:

**1.** Discomforts
– Ankle edema

– Dizziness

– False labor

– Family dynamics

– Fatigue

– Gingivitis

– Insomnia

– Leg cramps

– Perineal pressure

– Psychosocial responses

– Shortness of breath

– Urinary frequency

**2.** Self Care
– Baby preparation

– Exercise

– Labor preparation

– Nutrition

– Rest and relaxation

– Sexuality

**3.** Warning or Danger Signs
– Bleeding

– Burning on urination

– Chills and fever

– Diarrhea

– Epigastric pain

– Generalized edema

– Preterm labor

– Rupture of membranes

– Severe headache

– Visual disturbances

**Well-being assessments** of the mother and fetus involve physical assessment, laboratory tests, and fetal growth data collection. The purpose is to document pregnancy growth and development and to identify potential problems early. The following assessments are made during subsequent prenatal visits:

**Physical Assessment:**
- Maternal weight gain
- Maternal vital signs
- Fetal heart rate (120-160 bpm)
  - doppler auscultation from 10 or 12 weeks to 20 weeks
  - fetoscope auscultation from 19 or 20 weeks to birth
- Edema
- CVA tenderness
- Homan's sign

**Laboratory Tests:**
- Urinalysis (each visit)
- Hemoglobin and hematocrit (at 28 weeks)
- Blood glucose screen (at 24-28 weeks)
- Repeat Rh antibody screen for Rh negative mother (at 28 weeks)

**Fetal Growth and Development:**
- Maternal serum alpha-fetoprotein (at 15-18 weeks)
- Quickening (date of maternal perception of first movement)
- Fetal movement (maternal report and examiner palpation)
- Fundal height (at each visit)
- Fetal presentation (from 32 weeks to birth)

Assessment data are evaluated at each prenatal visit to determine whether or not the data indicate "normal" pregnancy progression or a potential problem. Weight gain is evaluated for an average weight gain of about 1 pound per week during the second and third trimesters and an average cumulative weight gain for the pregnancy of 25-35 pounds. The average fundal height assessment for the second and third trimesters is about 1 centimeter per week.

The data are evaluated for potential problems. For example, a mother who shows a weight gain of 10 pounds in one month and glycosuria may be developing gestational diabetes or she may be consuming a large amount of simple sugar foods/fluids. A 24-hour diet recall and blood glucose screen would be additional assessments to be made. Another example would be the mother who has gained 6 pounds in one week, has 2+ edema or greater, shows proteinuria greater than a "trace," and has an elevation in blood pressure of at least 30/15 mm Hg above her "normal" blood pressure. The assessment data would indicate development of PIH. Presence of proteinuria alone or in combination with dysuria and/or perineal itching could indicate a urinary tract or vaginal infection.

## Progressive Risk Assessment

At each prenatal visit, data are collected and evaluated from the episodic histories, physical assessment, laboratory tests, and psychological and emotional assessments to determine the risk status of the mother and fetus. In addition, progressive risk assessment procedures are scheduled to help identify potential risk for problems. For example, the MSAFP screens for fetal neural tube defects and is scheduled to be drawn at 15-18 weeks with maternal permission. The blood glucose screen is scheduled at 24-28 weeks to identify potential risk for gestational diabetes. Amniocentesis for chromosomal studies is recommended for mothers aged 35 or older to determine karyotype for diagnosing Down Syndrome in the fetus. When data indicate a potential change in risk status, additional screening and/or diagnostic procedures are performed to diagnose or rule out problems. Early intervention reduces the impact of complications of pregnancy and maternal and fetal problems.

# FETAL ASSESSMENT

Fetal assessment procedures that are in addition to the above "usual" or routine assessments made throughout the pregnancy may be required when the data do not support indications for fetal well-being. Several procedures can be performed depending on the potential problem and perceived severity of alteration in fetal well-being. The procedures can be classified as non-invasive and invasive. A summary of the procedures are as follows:

## Non-invasive Fetal Assessment Procedures

Non-invasive fetal assessment procedures include daily fetal movement counts, abdominal ultrasound, magnetic resonance imaging, biophysical profile, non-stress testing, and nipple stimulation stress testing. The procedures provide information regarding diagnosis of pregnancy (including the number of gestational sacs or fetuses in multiple gestation), gestational age, fetal growth, placental support, anomalies, and fetal well-being. A summary of each procedure follows:

1. **Daily Fetal Movement Counts** assess the number of fetal movements in a specified period of time. The assessment is performed by the expectant mother. At least 5-6 fetal movements in 30 minutes is desired.

The daily fetal movement count can be used by the low-risk mother two times a day, morning and evening. It is recommended for the high-risk mother three times daily, after each meal. If the mother does not count at least 5-6 movements in 30 minutes, she continues the count for 1 hour or more. Fewer than 3 fetal movements in 1 hour or fewer than 10 movements in 12 hours are indications for further assessment. In addition maternal perception of cessation of fetal movement for 12 hours at any time regardless of risk classification is an indication for further fetal well-being assessment (usually by non-stress testing).

2. **Abdominal Ultrasound** is the use of high frequency sound waves to produce static and/or dynamic images of the fetus (as well as other tissues and organs). It is used to diagnose pregnancy, confirm the number of fetuses, determine viability of the fetus, assess fetal gestational age, identify uterine abnormalities, measure amniotic fluid amount, evaluate fetal growth patterns, identify fetal anomalies, estimate fetal weight, visualize fetal heart and breathing movements, document placental location, and determine placental maturity.

3. **Magnetic Resonance Imaging** uses radio waves to produce images of soft tissue in multiple planes. It is used to evaluate fetal structure, systems, and organs; determine placental position, density, and disease processes; measure amniotic fluid amount; evaluate maternal soft tissue structure; evaluate the biochemical status of soft tissues and organs; and identify functional or metabolic malformations of soft tissues.

4. **Biophysical Profile** assesses fetal well-being by evaluating several biophysical parameters using electronic fetal monitoring and ultrasound to determine fetal status. Parameters include fetal breathing movements, gross fetal body movements, fetal tone, fetal heart rate reactivity, and amniotic fluid volume. Each parameter is evaluated according to specific criteria and given a score of 0 or 2. The maximum score is 10 and a score of 8-10, where amniotic fluid volume is normal, is considered desirable and indicates fetal well-being.

5. **Non-stress Testing** uses external electronic fetal monitoring to determine fetal heart rate response to fetal movement. Specifically, the reactive NST reveals at least 2 occurrences of fetal movement in a 20-minute period with a corresponding acceleration in the fetal heart rate (FHR) of at least 15 beats per minute lasting for at least 15 seconds. In addition, the baseline rate should be normal (120-160 bpm) and long-term variability should be average (see **Figure 2**). Reactive test results are desirable and indicate that if the fetus were born within a few days of the reactive test results, the fetus would be born in good condition.

Unsatisfactory or inconclusive NST test results indicate that less than 1 FHR acceleration occurred in 20 minutes, or the acceleration was less than 15 bpm and lasted less than 15 seconds and the long-term variability was less than average. Another reason for unsatisfactory or inconclusive test results is that the quality of the FHR tracing is inadequate for interpretation.

Nonreactive test results are not desirable and indicate that FHR accelerations did not occur with fetal movement (see **Figure 3**). Because nonreactive test results do not identify the fetus who is at risk for hypoxia, nonreactive NST results should be followed by further evaluation (contraction stress test, BPP, amniotic fluid index).

**Note:** Electronic Fetal Monitoring (EFM) permits collection of data to determine fetal well-being, fetal response to stimulation (uterine contractions, fetal movement), and occurrence, frequency, duration, and intensity (with internal EFM) of uterine contractions. The following terms are used in describing and evaluating EFM data:

    a. **FHR Baseline** is the average fetal heart rate determined between uterine contractions and fetal movements over a 10-minute period (see **Figure 4**). A desirable rate is 120-160 bpm.

    b. **Bradycardia** is a FHR of less than 120 bpm over a 10-minute period (see **Figure 5**).

    c. **Tachycardia** is a FHR of greater than 160 bpm over a 10-minute period (see **Figure 6**).

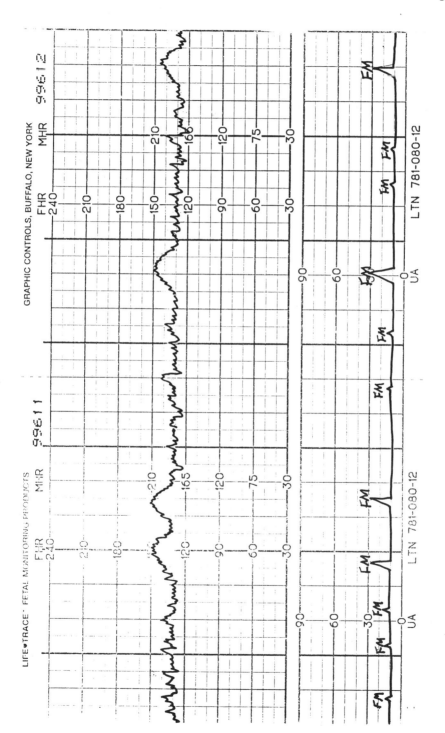

**Figure 2.** Reactive Non-Stress Test (NST). FHR accelerations of at least 15 bpm lasting at least 15 seconds occur with fetal movement (FM).

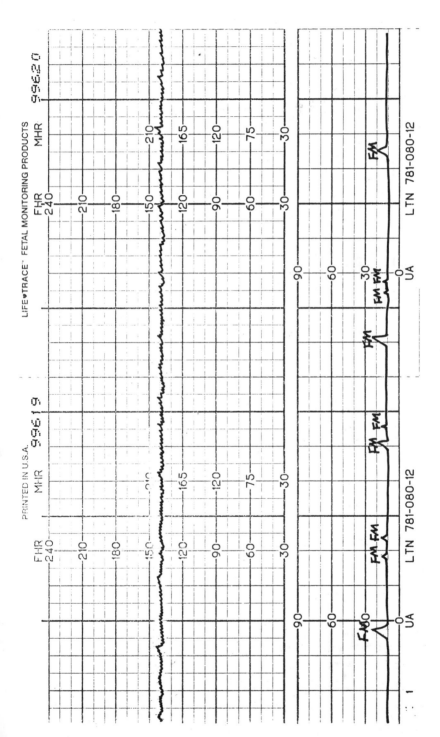

**Figure 3.** Nonreactive Non-stress Test. Fetal movement (FM) occur with no FHR accelerations.

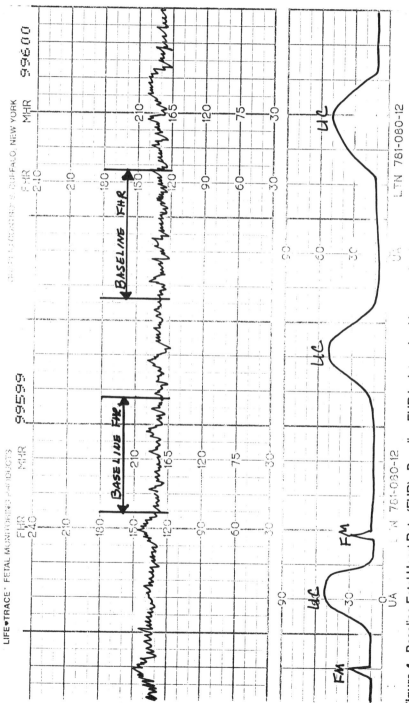

**Figure 4.** Baseline Fetal Heart Rate (FHR). Baseline FHR is determined between fetal stimulations, fetal movement (FM) and uterine contractions (UC).

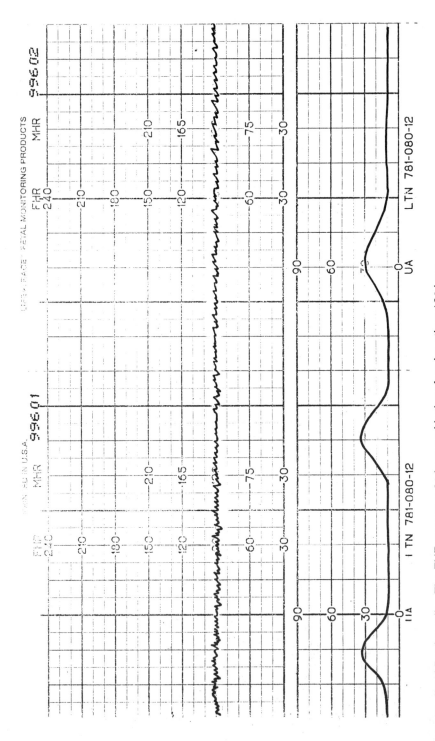

**Figure 5.** Fetal Bradycardia. The FHR averages 90 bpm and is therefore less than 120 bpm.

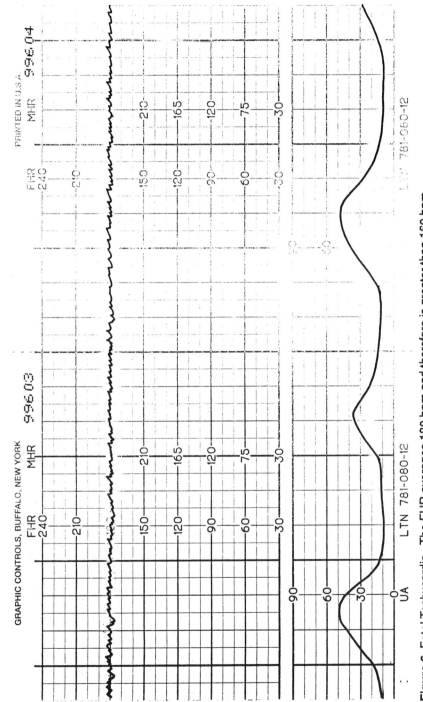

**Figure 6.** Fetal Tachycardia. The FHR averages 180 bpm and therefore is greater than 160 bpm.

**d. Baseline variability** is the irregularity of the FHR tracing that indicates a balance of stimulation of the heart by the sympathetic and parasympathetic nervous systems.

Baseline variability is described in terms of both short-term (STV) and long-term variability (LTV). LTV can be evaluated from the EFM strip in both external and internal mode. STV can only be evaluated accurately in internal mode.

**STV** is the change in FHR from one heartbeat to the next and is also called beat-to-beat variability. It is evaluated as being present or absent (see **Figures 7 and 8**).

**LTV** is the change in FHR baseline over time. It is evaluated by both the number of cycles of change per minute and by the number of FHR beats per minute for each cycle (see **Figures 7 and 8**). The number of cycles of change per minute desired is 2-6. The number of fetal heartbeats per minute is evaluated according to the following:

| | |
|---|---|
| No Variability: | 0-2 bpm |
| Minimal Variability: | 3-5 bpm |
| Average Variability: | 6-10 bpm |
| Moderate Variability: | 11-25 bpm |
| Marked Variability: | >25 bpm |

STV and LTV usually vary together. Thus, if LTV is average, STV is usually present. If LTV is absent, STV is usually absent, too.

**e. Accelerations** are temporary increases in the FHR from the baseline in response to stimulation, most often fetal movement and uterine contractions (see **Figure 9**). Accelerations are indicative of fetal well-being.

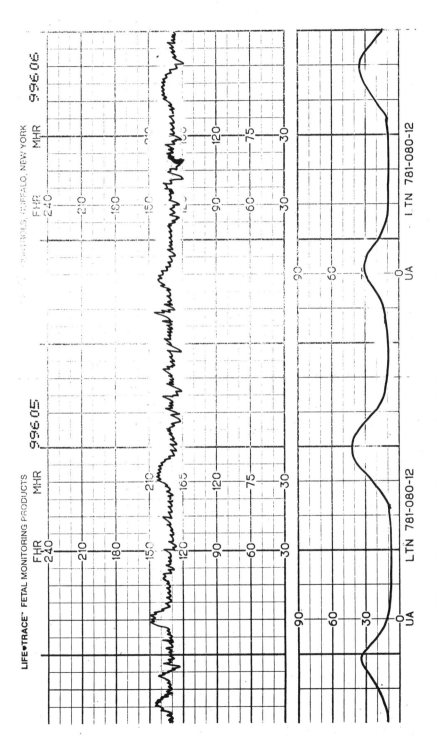

**Figure 7.** Short-term (STV) and Long-term (LTV) Variability. STV is present and LTV is average.

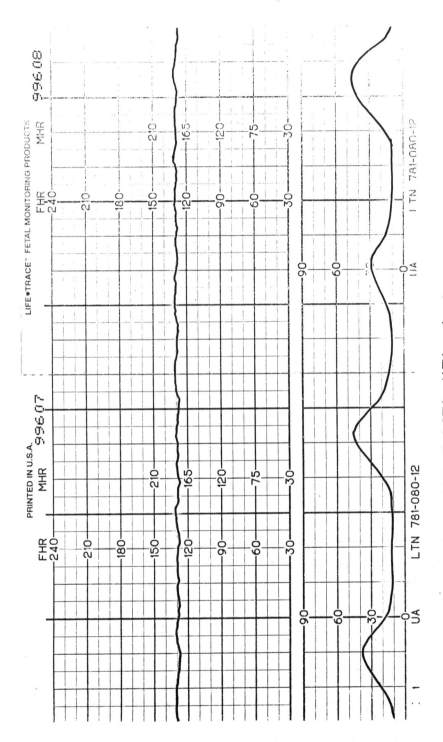

**Figure 8.** Short-term and Long-term Variability. Both STV and LTV are absent.

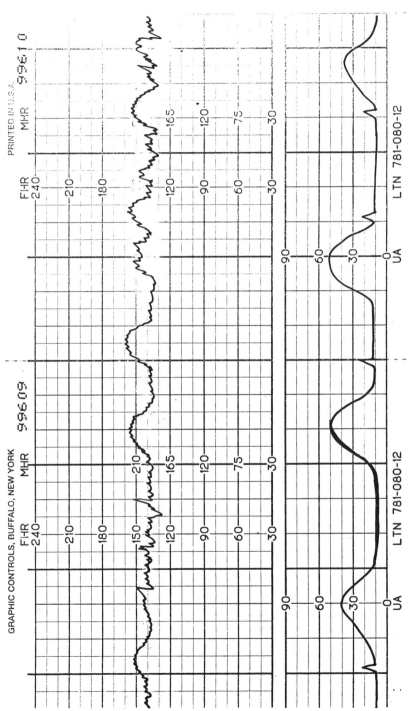

**Figure 9.** FHR Acceleration. The FHR acclerates in response to FM and UCs.

f. **Decelerations** are temporary decreases in the FHR from the baseline in response to stimulation or decreased oxygen availability. They are classified as early, late, or variable. Decelerations may be interpreted as being benign or non-reassuring depending on the type. The type of deceleration is determined by the waveform and the time at which they occur in relation to uterine contractions. Thus, decelerations are usually noted during labor or contraction stress testing.

**Early Decelerations** have a waveform that is uniform and inversely "mirrors" the uterine contraction with the nadir (low point) of the deceleration occurring during the peak of the uterine contraction. The onset of the early deceleration is before the peak of the uterine contraction and the recovery (return of FHR to baseline) is by the end of the uterine contraction (see **Figure 10**). Early decelerations are caused by pressure on the fetal head and are considered benign.

**Late Decelerations** have a uniform waveform that "mirrors" the uterine contraction with the nadir occurring after the peak of the contraction. The onset of the late deceleration is at or after the peak of the contraction and the recovery is after the end of the contraction (see **Figure 11**). Late decelerations are caused by placental insufficiency, indicate decreased fetal oxygen transfer, and are considered non-reassuring.

**Variable Decelerations** have a variable waveform usually with sharp decreases and increases. The onset of the variable deceleration is abrupt and varies in relation to the uterine contraction pattern and the recovery is usually rapid (see **Figure 12)**. The variable deceleration is often preceded and followed by accelerations called "shoulders." The appearance of shoulders is considered reassuring. The occurrence of one acceleration only occurring as the variable deceleration returns to FHR baseline is called an "overshoot" and is considered non-reassuring. Variable decelerations are caused by umbilical cord compression. They are frequently observed in association with maternal pushing efforts in the second stage of labor.

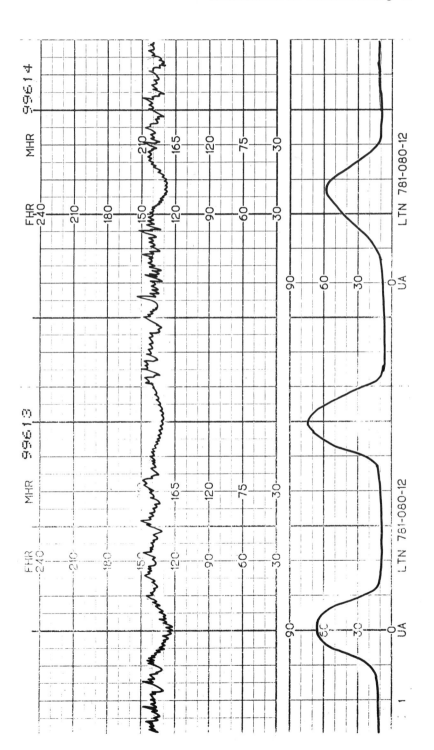

**Figure 10.** Early Decelerations. The nadir of the deceleration occurs at the peak of the UC.

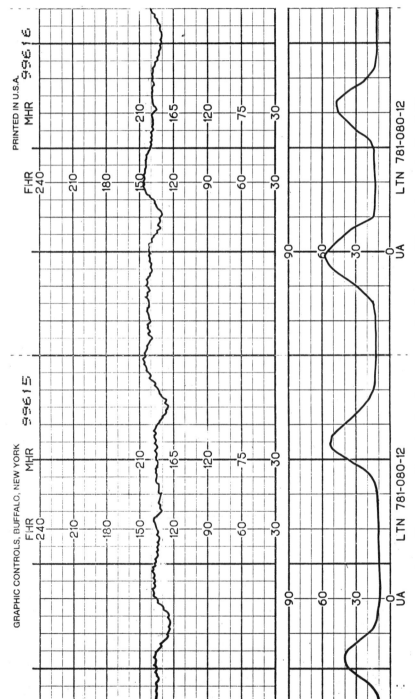

**Figure 11.** Late Decelerations. The onset of late decelerations occurs after the peak of the uterine contraction (UC).

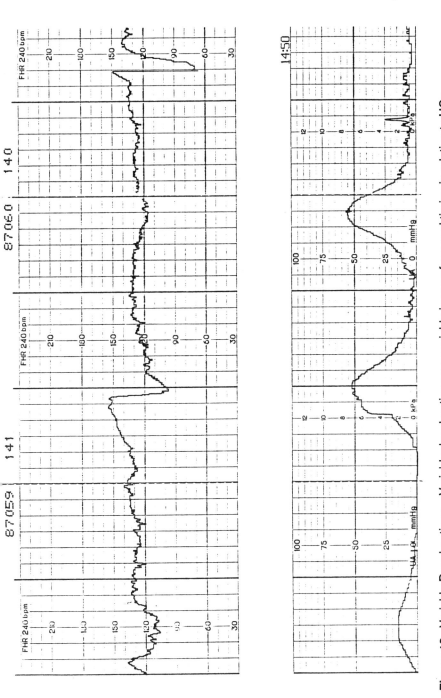

**Figure 12. Variable Decelerations.** Variable decelerations are variable in waveform and timing in relation to UCs. Note the presence of "shoulders."

6. **Nipple-stimulation stress testing** is one form of stress test of the fetus. Stress tests introduce stress on the fetus in the form of uterine contractions to identify the fetus who is stable at rest but experiences hypoxia during uterine contractions because of decreased placental perfusion. Stress testing is called Contraction Stress Test (CST). Contractions can be caused by oxytocin production in response to nipple stimulation.

The **CST** evaluates the capability of the placenta to transfer oxygen to the fetus and remove carbon dioxide. The CST requires the occurrence of 3 uterine contractions of good quality (at least 40 seconds duration and palpable to the examiner) in a 10-minute period.

A negative test result is desirable and indicates that 3 uterine contractions of good quality occurred in 10 minutes with NO LATE DECELERATIONS (see **Figure 13**). In addition, the baseline variability is usually average, and if fetal movements occur, FHR accelerations are present. Negative results indicate that the fetus is well at the time of the testing and will not need additional testing for 7 days.

A positive test result is not desirable and indicates that persistent late decelerations occurred or late decelerations occurred with at least 50% of the uterine contractions (see **Figure 14**). Late decelerations may indicate insufficient respiratory reserve of the placenta and fetal hypoxia. Thus, positive test results indicate increased risk of perinatal morbidity and mortality.

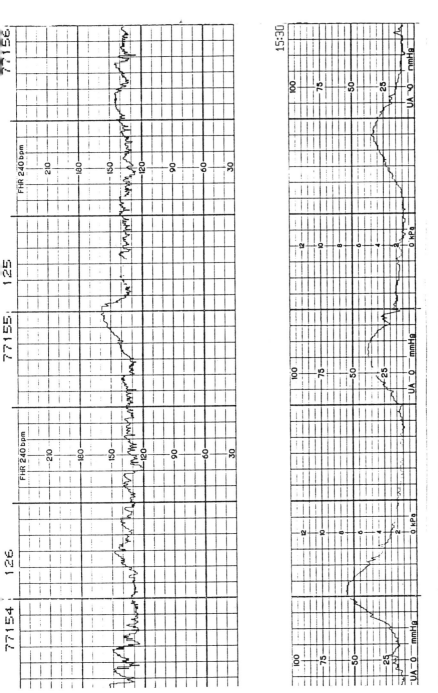

**Figure 13.** Negative Contraction Stress Test (CST). Adequate UCs in terms of frequency, duration, and intensity occurred and there are no late decelerations and baseline variability is average.

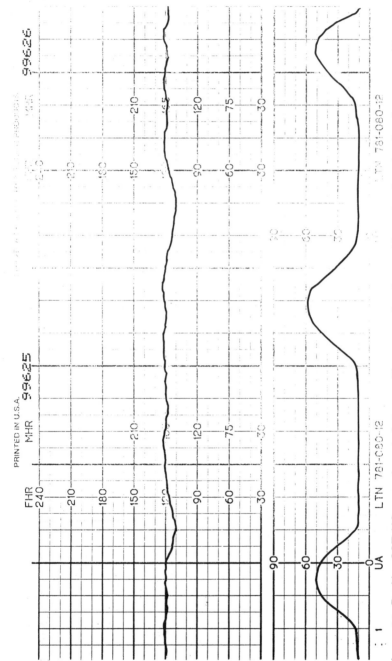

**Figure 14.** Positive CST. UCs are adequate in terms of frequency, duration, and intensity; late decelerations occur with more than 50% of the UCs; and baseline variability is absent .

**Suspicious or equivocal test** results indicate that late decelerations occurred with less than 50% of the uterine contractions. The CST is repeated a few hours later or the next day.

**Hyperstimulation** results occur when the uterine frequency is less than 2 minutes, the duration is greater than 90 seconds, and/or the tone is hypertonic.

**Unsatisfactory test** results indicate the uterine contraction pattern and/or the tracing was inadequate for interpretation.

## Invasive Fetal Assessment Procedures

Invasive fetal assessment procedures include oxytocin challenge test (OCT), amniocentesis, percutaneous umbilical blood sampling, chorionic villi sampling, and MSAFP. The procedures provide information about fetal maturity, placental support, gestational age, anomalies, fetal anemia, and fetal well-being. A summary of each procedure is as follows:

1. **Oxytocin Challenge Test** is the second type of CST and is considered invasive because exogenous intravenous oxytocin administration is required to stimulate the 3 uterine contractions of good quality in a 10-minute period. OCT results are evaluated the same as the nipple stimulation CST (see CST results).

2. **Amniocentesis** is the transabdominal insertion of a needle into the amniotic sac through the uterus and withdrawal of amniotic fluid for evaluation. Needle insertion is accomplished with the aid of ultrasound visualization to locate adequate pockets of amniotic fluid and to avoid insertion through the placenta or into the fetus. Indications for amniocentesis include genetic evaluation, fetal sex and maturity determination, presence of neural tube defect (alpha-fetoprotein level), and presence of intrauterine infection.

   Lecithin/sphingomyelin (L/S) ratios, phosphatidylglycerol levels, bilirubin levels, creatinine levels, lipid cell presence, and presence of bacteria and meconium in the amniotic fluid can be determined from the amniotic fluid. In addition, chromosome studies can be completed from fetal cells present in the fluid. There is a very slight risk of adverse outcome, such as rupture of the membranes, preterm labor, or infection, as a result of the procedure.

3. **Percutaneous Umbilical Blood Sampling** is transabdominal insertion of a needle into the umbilical vein vessel through the uterus to obtain a fetal blood sample for analysis. Needle insertion is accomplished under the guidance of ultrasound. The blood sample is used for determining CBC, fetal blood type, direct Coomb's, level of maternal drugs in the fetus, fetal metabolic disorders, blood gases, karyotyping, acid-base status for intrauterine growth retarded fetuses, detection of infection, and intrauterine transfusion for fetuses with isoimmune hemolytic

anemia. Complications are unusual and are due to leaking of blood from the puncture site, rupture of membranes, intrauterine infection, and fetal bradycardia.

4. **Chorionic Villus Sampling** is the transcervical insertion of a needle into the fetal portion of the placenta between 10 and 12 weeks to evaluate the genetic makeup of the fetus. The advantage of chorionic villus sampling is that it can be performed early so that first trimester abortion can be accomplished for fetuses with genetic defect(s). A disadvantage of performing chorionic villus sampling between 8 and 9.5 weeks is a risk of fetal limb defect occurrence.

5. **Maternal Serum Alpha-fetoprotein** (MSAFP) is used as a screening test for neural tube defects. Maternal serum levels of alpha-fetoprotein (AFP) are determined between 15 and 18 weeks gestation. If maternal serum levels are elevated, ultrasound can be used to confirm the diagnosis of neural tube defect and/or AFP levels in the amniotic fluid are determined by amniocentesis to confirm the diagnosis of neural tube defect in the fetus.

Indications for performing the additional assessment procedures include:

1. Presence of Chronic Maternal Disease
   - Hypertension
   - Diabetes mellitus
   - Cyanotic heart disease
   - Hyperthyroidism
   - Lupus
2. Occurrence of Pregnancy Complications
   - PIH
   - Gestational diabetes
   - Preterm labor or history of previous preterm labor
   - Rh isoimmunization
   - Intrauterine growth retardation
   - Postterm pregnancy
   - History of fetal demise
   - Abruptio placentae or placenta previa
   - Maternal infection
   - History of chromosomal or genetic disorder
   - Hydramnios
   - Oligohydramnios
   - FHR arrythmias
   - Elevated MSAFP

# CHAPTER 5

# NURSING INTERVENTION

*Nursing intervention for expectant mothers involves education for self-care, health promotion, and health maintenance, as well as intervention for alterations in health. Interventions for alterations in health of mother and fetus are included in the discussion of Selected Prenatal Complications.*

## EDUCATION FOR SELF-CARE

**Education for self-care** includes counseling for coping with the "minor discomforts of pregnancy." In general, the discomforts experienced by the expectant mother can be categorized by trimester.

**First trimester discomforts** commonly include nausea and/or vomiting, breast tenderness, urinary frequency, fatigue, mood swings, increased vaginal discharge (leukorrhea), and nasal stuffiness. Counseling for each discomfort involves explaining the cause(s) and self-care measures which are summarized below:

1. **Nausea and/or vomiting** may occur at any time during the day even though it is commonly called "morning sickness." Intervention incorporates explanation for potential cause (hormone levels, effect of hormones, hypoglycemia, hypotension) and self-care measures to reduce or prevent the occurrence. Self-care measures that are recommended are six small high protein and complex carbohydrate meals per day, ingestion of dry carbohydrate before arising followed soon after arising by protein, alternating solid ("dry") and fluid ("wet") intake, ingesting a source of protein at the time the expectant mother is awake for nightly "trips to the bathroom," and avoiding fried, fatty, gas-forming, or spicy foods. If the expectant mother is vomiting several times daily or shows signs of dehydration, she is instructed to contact her primary health care provider.

2. **Breast tenderness** occurs in response to hormone stimulation. Self-care involves wearing a supportive bra that has wide non-elastic straps, cups that are large enough to contain the entire breast, and expandable capabilities for increasing chest circumference. The mother may find that wearing a supportive bra even at night provides increased comfort. She may also position pillows above and below the breasts to prevent the breasts from resting on the bed in the prone position.

3. **Urinary frequency** in the first trimester is due to the pressure of the enlarging uterus on the bladder. Relief is experienced in the second trimester when the uterus becomes an abdominal organ. Self-care measures include reducing late evening fluid intake

while maintaining daily water intake of 8-10 glasses. Suggest that the mother use the nocturnal urination occurrences to maintain her blood glucose level by ingesting protein while she is "up." Remind her that nocturia is "normal" and will end at approximately 12 weeks. Review signs of dysuria and the recommendation to contact her primary health care provider if urinary frequency is accompanied by dysuria.

4. **Fatigue** may be caused by changes in hormone levels and is thought to be protective. Self-care measures include adequate nighttime rest (8-10 hours), daily rest periods, and balanced nutritional intake to avoid anemia.

5. **Mood swings** are common during pregnancy and are thought to be due to hormone changes and developmental adaptations precipitated by the pregnancy. Self-care measures include identification of need for and acceptance of support by partner, family, and friends.

6. **Leukorrhea** occurs in response to hormonal stimulated changes of the cervix and vagina. Self-care measures include hygiene (but NO DOUCHING OR VAGINAL DEODORANTS), wearing cotton panties, and avoiding tight fitting jeans/pants. Remind the mother to report signs of vaginal infection (yellow or green discharge, odorous discharge, itching, external dysuria) to her primary health care provider.

7. **Nasal stuffiness** occurs in response to high estrogen levels. Self-care measures include use of a cool-air humidifier. Remind the mother to avoid the use of nasal sprays or decongestants.

**Second trimester discomforts** commonly include backache, carpal tunnel syndrome, constipation, flatulence, food cravings, heartburn, round ligament pain, supine hypotension, and varicose veins. Nursing intervention for the second trimester discomforts also includes explanation for the cause(s), self-care measures, and reminders to report danger signs to the primary health care provider.

1. **Backache** is caused primarily by the shift in center of gravity as the pregnancy progresses. Self-care measures include maintaining good body alignment, use of body mechanics, wearing low heeled shoes, use of the pelvic rock (pelvic tilt) exercise, and asking for a backrub.

2. **Carpal tunnel syndrome** is caused by compression of the median nerve as it passes through the carpal tunnel. Self-care measures include avoiding repetitive hand motions, elevating the affected hand, and use of splinting of the affected hand to maintain the wrist in the neutral position.

3. **Constipation** is caused by the impact of progesterone on the GI tract, iron supplement, and pressure of the enlarging uterus. Self-care measures include avoiding fatty and gas-forming meals,

consuming smaller more frequent meals, increasing fluid and roughage intake, scheduling time for regular elimination, and increasing exercise such as walking. Remind the mother to avoid use of laxatives without specific recommendations by her primary health care provider.

4. **Flatulence** is caused by decreased gastrointestinal tract motility (progesterone), pressure of the enlarging uterus, and air swallowing. Self-care measures include avoidance of gas-forming and fatty foods, simple carbohydrates, chewing food thoroughly, consuming smaller, more frequent meals, increasing exercise (walking), and maintaining regular bowel habits.

5. **Food cravings** may be experienced by expectant mothers. The cause is unknown. Self-care measures include maintaining consumption of a balanced, nutritious diet. As long as food cravings do not include consumption of nonfood substances or interfere with consumption of a balanced diet, the cravings may be satisfied. Remind the mother to report craving of nonfood substances to her primary health care provider.

6. **Heartburn** is caused by the effect of progesterone on the GI tract and the pressure of the enlarging uterus resulting in regurgitation of stomach contents into the esophagus. Self-care measures include avoiding fried and fatty foods, consuming smaller, more frequent meals, avoiding the supine position for 2 hours following a meal, maintaining good posture, and sipping milk or hot tea or chewing gum to relieve discomfort temporarily. Maalox may be recommended, but baking soda and Alka-Seltzer should be avoided to prevent electrolyte imbalance due to sodium content.

7. **Round ligament pain** is caused by stretching of the ligament by the enlarging uterus. Self-care measures include avoiding over-stretching by use of good body mechanics; resting, squatting or drawing legs up close to the abdomen; applying a warm heating pad, rubbing or placing the hand over the area of discomfort (warmth); and taking a warm bath.

8. **Supine hypotension** is caused by pressure of the enlarging uterus on the ascending vena cava in the supine position. Self-care measures include avoiding the supine position, using the side-lying position with the legs flexed and upper leg supported for comfort, and using the semi-sitting position. Remind the mother that placental and renal perfusion is reduced in the supine position.

9. **Varicose veins** are caused by the effect of hormones, pressure of the enlarging uterus, and hereditary influence. Varicose veins may occur in the legs, anal area (hemorrhoids), or vulvar area. Self-care measures include avoiding prolonged periods of standing or sitting, avoiding constrictive clothing, avoiding straining with

bowel movements, avoiding crossing the legs, wearing support hose, elevating the legs frequently, walking around periodically to promote venous return, elevating hips for vulvar and anal varicosities, and use of warm sitz baths and astringent compresses for vulvar and anal varicosities.

**Third trimester discomforts** commonly include the discomforts identified for the second trimester plus ankle edema, faintness, insomnia, leg cramps, shortness of breath, and urinary frequency and urgency. As with the first and second trimester discomforts, causes and self-care need to be explained to the expectant mother.

1. **Ankle edema** is caused by the hormonal effect and pressure of the enlarging uterus that reduce venous return from the lower extremities. Self-care includes avoiding prolonged sitting or standing, avoiding constrictive clothing, avoiding the supine position, drinking 8-10 glasses of water daily to promote the natural excretion of fluid, wearing support hose, and resting with the legs and hips elevated. Remind the mother that edema of the hands and face (generalized) are not a minor discomfort of pregnancy but a potential danger sign, especially when accompanied by visual changes, headache, and oliguria.

2. **Faintness** in the third trimester is usually caused by postural hypotension. Self-care measures include avoiding sudden position changes, avoiding standing for prolonged periods of time, avoiding orthostatic hypotension and supine hypotension, and sitting down with her head between her legs or lying down when she feels faint.

3. **Insomnia** often occurs for the same reasons it occurs in non-pregnant women, plus exaggerated fetal movements, the occurrence of muscle cramps, the inability to find a comfortable position because of the enlarging uterus, shortness of breath, and urinary frequency. Self-help measures include taking a warm shower, drinking warm milk or a warm noncaffeine beverage, asking for a back rub, using pillows to support the back and extremities, using deep breathing and relaxation techniques, and avoiding stimulating activities near bedtime. Remind the mother to avoid sleep medication without a recommendation from her primary health care provider.

4. **Leg cramps** may be caused by pressure of the enlarging uterus on nerves supplying the lower extremities, an imbalance of the calcium/phosphorus ratio, fatigue, reduced peripheral circulation, and pointing the toes when extending the leg. Self-care measures include asking someone to place pressure on the knee while dorsiflexing the foot, standing and leaning forward on the extended affected leg, avoiding pointing the toes, and recom-

mending aluminum hydroxide gel to absorb phosphorus. Remember to evaluate Homan's sign to rule out the presence of a blood clot.

5. **Shortness of breath** is caused by pressure on the diaphragm by the enlarging uterus. Lightening improves this discomfort. Self-care measures include avoiding large meals and use of pillows for comfort at night or during rest periods. Remember to assess the mother for anemia or asthma.

6. **Urinary urgency and frequency** is caused by pressure of the presenting part after lightening. Self-care measures for urinary frequency are the same as for the first trimester. Self-care measures for urinary urgency include Kegel exercises.

# EDUCATION FOR HEALTH PROMOTION

**Education for health promotion** involves teaching self-care and life-style behaviors to prevent complications of pregnancy and to promote optimal well-being for pregnancy and beyond. Health promotion education includes prevention of urinary tract infection (UTI) and sexually-transmitted diseases, prevention of cystocele, substance use, exercise, rest and sleep, nutrition, sexual relations, relaxation, and parenting and childbirth education.

1. **UTI** has been linked to stimulation of preterm labor. Thus, prevention is essential. Prevention measures include:

   a. Drinking 8-10 glasses of water daily to prevent urine stasis;

   b. Drinking cranberry juice daily to discourage bacteria growth by lowering the pH of the urinary tract;

   c. Wiping from front to back to prevent transfer of bacteria from the perianal area to the periurethral area;

   D. Using white, unperfumed, soft, good quality toilet paper to prevent irritation;

   e. Wearing cotton crotch panties and pantyhose to reduce the amount of heat and moisture trapped in the perineal area and thus reduce the potential for bacteria growth;

   f. Avoiding tight jeans and pants to prevent trapping heat and moisture in the perineal area;

   g. Urinating frequently and especially before sleeping to prevent bacterial growth due to prolonged urine retention; and

   h. Urinating following sexual intercourse to eliminate bacteria introduced during intercourse.

2. **Vaginal infection** can be due to change in vaginal flora or due to sexually-transmitted diseases (STD's). Preventive measures include:

   a. Keeping the perineal area dry to prevent bacterial growth (similar measures for preventing UTI);

   b. Consuming active-culture yogurt to maintain vaginal flora and prevent multiplication of yeast organisms, especially when taking antibiotics;

   c. Avoiding use of douches and vaginal/perineal deodorants;

   d. Maintaining a monogamous relationship to prevent transfer of STDs and/or using condoms.

3. **Cystocele** is relaxation of the anterior vaginal wall with corresponding prolapse of the bladder into the area of relaxation. Preventive measures include emptying the bladder when the urge occurs and practicing Kegel exercises several times daily (to strengthen the pubococcygeus muscle and enhance support to the pelvic organs).

4. **Substance use** (alcohol, tobacco, marijuana, heroin, cocaine) is harmful for the mother and embryo/fetus during pregnancy and the mother and infant/child after birth. Preventive measures include abstinence and education regarding the pregnancy and life-long detrimental effects of substance use.

5. **Exercise** during pregnancy is primarily focused on health and comfort during pregnancy. The exercises for pregnancy include the following:

   a. Partial sit-ups to strengthen the abdominal muscles;

   b. The pelvic tilt/rock to prevent back strain and reduce backache;

   c. Kegel exercises to strengthen the pubococcygeus muscle;

   d. Tailor sitting to stretch the pelvic floor muscles for birth and to strengthen the thigh muscles;

   e. Squatting to stretch the pelvic floor muscles for birth; and

   f. Walking, swimming, or cycling to improve muscle tone.

   **Note:** Remind the expectant mother to avoid exercises that might put her at risk for falls or loss of balance.

   Life-long exercises include continuation of partial sit-ups, pelvic tilt/rock, Kegel exercises, and walking (as a weight-bearing exercise to prevent osteoporosis and as a cardiovascular exercise to promote cardiac reserve).

6. **Rest and sleep** are required for physical and emotional well-being. Expectant mothers tend to become tired easily during the first and third trimesters especially. Preventive measures include adequate rest at night (8-10 hours) and scheduling short rest periods during the day.

7. **Nutrition** is important throughout life and is essential for preventing low birth weight neonates. The average weight gain desired for the expectant mother is 25-35 pounds distributed across the three trimesters of pregnancy. In general, the fetus is at risk for intrauterine growth retardation if the mother has not gained at least 10 pounds by 20 weeks gestation.

   The appropriate weight gain for each individual expectant mother can be determined by using the Body Mass Index (BMI). The BMI is calculated by dividing the mother's weight in kilograms by the square of her height in meters. The BMI determines whether she is underweight and will need to gain 28-40 pounds, normal weight and will need to gain the average 25-35 pounds, or overweight and will need to gain 15-25 pounds.

   Maternal weight gain must come from a balanced diet rather than high calorie and limited nutrient foods. Using the Food Pyramid as a teaching aid shows the expectant mother the foods, and the number of servings per day, recommended. Establishing good nutritional habits in pregnancy can be extended to life-long family habits.

   Specific nutrients that are increased in pregnancy include the minerals calcium and phosphorus, iron, iodine, and magnesium. Also included are zinc, protein, the fat-soluble vitamins D and E, and the water-soluble vitamins B-complex (especially folic acid) and C. With selection of the recommended number of servings from each of the Food Pyramid groups all of the requirements can be met, except for iron which is usually supplemented during pregnancy. If the mother is lactose intolerant, she may need to use lactase-treated milk, take lactase tablets before consuming dairy products, or use calcium supplements.

   Cultural, religious, and family preferences need to be incorporated in planning balanced meals. Remember to assess for the practice of pica (ingestion of nonfood substances) by expectant mothers. Current recommendations also suggest avoiding, or at least, limiting intake of caffeine and artificial sweeteners.

8. **Sexual relations** are considered safe throughout an uncomplicated pregnancy. Sexual activity needs to be avoided if bleeding or rupture of the membranes occurs. As pregnancy progresses, the mother may experience a change in desire for sexual activity and alternative positions may be more comfortable. Recommendations include side-by-side, female superior, or vaginal rear

entry as positions to avoid discomfort, shortness of breath, or supine hypotension. In addition, nonsexual intercourse activities such as cuddling and kissing may be substituted for sexual intercourse.

9. **Relaxation** may include time out for reflecting on favorite places and events and slow deep breathing exercises in addition to actual rest and sleep. Such "mini-vacations" during the day or during stressful periods relax tense muscles and increase oxygen levels during pregnancy and life-long.

10. **Parenting and childbirth education** provides group learning and individual practice of breathing and relaxation techniques for labor and birth, decision-making for labor and birth, care of the postpartum mother and the newborn, preparation for the chosen method of feeding the newborn, and identification of expectations for the birthing experience and early postpartum period.

Infant breast feeding preparation should include careful assessment of maternal breasts for identification of inverted nipples. Measures to correct inverted nipples need to be initiated during the last trimester of pregnancy. Practicing Hoffman's exercises and wearing a nipple cup draw the nipple out so the neonate can grasp it.

# EDUCATION FOR HEALTH MAINTENANCE

**Health maintenance** education is initially applied to pregnancy and extended to include life-long benefits and recommendations. Pregnancy is a time when families seem motivated to change habits "for the baby" and can be assisted in establishing positive life-long health behaviors. Health maintenance education includes topics in health promotion education plus breast self exam, dental health, employment, immunizations, over-the-counter medications, and safety.

1. **Breast self exam (BSE)** remains the best method for early detection of breast lumps. Every woman needs to practice BSE at the same time every month so that she is very familiar with the texture of her breasts and can readily recognize any changes in texture to report to her primary health provider. Establishing the habit of monthly BSE during pregnancy will promote continuing the practice following pregnancy.

2. **Dental health** begins with consistent oral hygiene and includes regular dental checkups and balanced nutritional intake. Brushing at least twice daily, flossing at least once daily, and rinsing the mouth with cool water after consuming food or beverages promotes dental health.

3. **Employment** during pregnancy may cause undue stress and fatigue and may expose the expectant mother to teratogenic agents. Careful history, maternal assessment, and evaluation are required at each prenatal visit to determine the effect on maternal and fetal well-being.

   Combining mothering and employment activities requires careful life-long scheduling and planning. Planning for comfort, relaxation, and stress reduction techniques at work during pregnancy can help establish life-long patterns for use following pregnancy. In addition, scheduling realistic workloads for work and home during pregnancy will help the working mother continue the practice following pregnancy.

4. **Immunizations** with live or attenuated live viruses are contraindicated during pregnancy but those with killed viruses may be given and certain vaccines may be given prophylactally following exposure. Pregnancy is an optimal time to reinforce keeping maternal immunizations current and to emphasize the need for completing all recommended vaccines for the infant and child.

5. **Over-the-counter (OTC) medications** are contraindicated during pregnancy, especially during the first trimester. The expectant mother must consult her primary health provider before taking OTCs. In general, life-long habits should be established to limit use of OTCs and when deciding to use them, to select those that contain as few ingredients as possible rather than those with a mixture of ingredients (such as a decongestant, cough suppressant, antihistamine, anticholinergic, topical anesthetic).

6. **Safety** during pregnancy includes avoiding exposure to teratogenic agents and organisms, using seat belts, practicing good body mechanics, wearing industrial safety devices as recommended, reading all labels for products, and scheduling rest periods. Pregnancy is a good time to reinforce life-long safety habits and to emphasize safety requirements for the infant and child (such as car seats).

CHAPTER 6

# SELECTED PRENATAL COMPLICATIONS

*Prenatal complications can be placed into the category of disorders the expectant mother has when pregnancy occurs or the category of disorders that occur only during pregnancy. Complications that occur most commonly in each of the categories are summarized below.*

## PRE-EXISTING DISORDERS

**Preexisting disorders** that the expectant mother may be experiencing at the time pregnancy occurs include cardiac disease, diabetes mellitus, and genitourinary infections. The symptoms, consequences, assessment, and interventions for each disorder are summarized below:

1. **Cardiac disease is caused by myocardial disease, valvular** disease, or congenital defect. The severity of the disease is classified according to the degree of disability or presence of symptoms in relation to activity.

   There are four classes established by the New York Heart Asso-cia-tion. Class I means no symptoms occur at normal levels of activity. Class II means symptoms such as fatigue, shortness of breath, palpitations, or anginal pain occur with normal activity. Class III means symptoms occur with less than normal activity. Class IV means symptoms occur at rest. Limitation of activities range from no limitation for Class I mothers to limitation of all activities for Class IV mothers. Class II mothers have slight limitation of activities and Class III have moderate limitation.

   The expected outcome of the pregnancy is based on the class which is determined at the end of the first trimester and again at approximately 28 weeks. The greatest risk occurs when the blood volume peaks at approximately 28-32 weeks. Class I and II mothers can expect successful pregnancies and births. Class III mothers usually require bedrest (moderate limitation of activities) to complete pregnancy and birth. Class IV mothers are not good candidates for pregnancy.

   a. Symptoms of cardiac decompensation include the following:

      **Subjective:**

      – Fatigue

      – Difficulty breathing

- Smothering feeling

- Coughing

- Palpitations

- Swelling

**Objective:**

- Dyspnea

- Generalized edema

- Heart murmurs

- Tachypnea

- Tachycardia

- Crackles at the lung bases

- Moist, frequent cough

- Cyanosis (lips, nail beds)

   **b.** Consequences for the fetus include increased risk of spontaneous abortion, increased risk of preterm labor, and intrauterine growth retardation. Maternal consequences include increased risk for maternal morbidity and mortality.

   **c.** Assessment includes the routine pregnancy assessments plus assessment for anemia, symptoms of cardiac decompensation, undue emotional stress, and fetal growth.

   **d.** Intervention includes the usual pregnancy educational interventions provided for noncardiac mothers plus education regarding medications, scheduling more frequent assessment, nutrition counseling, weight gain, and planning rest periods and restriction of activities based on classification.

   Medications include prenatal vitamin and iron supplements, possible prophylactic antibiotics, possible anticoagulant therapy (Heparin), possible diuretic therapy, possible antiarrhythmic medication and Digitalis therapy.

**2. Diabetes mellitus is an endocrine disorder characterized by** alteration in protein, fat, carbohydrate, and insulin metabolism, and the progression of hypertensive disease. Diabetes mellitus is classified according to dependence on insulin except during pregnancy.

During pregnancy, diabetes mellitus is classified based on White's Classification which is based on age at diagnosis, duration of the disease in years, and the presence and type of hypertensive disorder. White's Class A includes chemical diabetes and gestational diabetes (see Gestational Disorders below) and involves no hypertensive disease. Class B includes women who were diagnosed at or after age 20, have had the disorder less than 10 years, usually are noninsulin dependent when not pregnant, and have no hypertensive disease. Class C can be divided into two categories and includes mothers who were diagnosed between age 10 and 19 or who have had the disorder for 10-19 years and have minimal vascular involvement. Class D has several categories dependent upon the progression of the vascular involvement. The mothers were diagnosed by age 10, have had the disorder 20 years or longer, and have beginning retinopathy, calcification of leg vessels, or hypertension. Class E is mothers with demonstration of calcified pelvic vessels on x-ray. Since x-ray is contraindicated in pregnancy, this classification is no longer used. Class F is the mother whose vascular involve- ment has progressed to the level of nephropathy. Class H includes the mother whose hypertensive disorder has progressed to include cardiopathy. Class R includes the mother whose hypertensive involvement has progressed to the level of prolifer- ating retinopathy. The Class T mother has experienced a renal transplant due to progression of the hypertensive involvement.

The outcome is dependent on maintaining blood sugar control and on the vascular involvement. In general, mothers in classes A, B, and C tend to have macrosomic infants while mothers in the other classes tend to have small for gestational age infants because of the impact of vascular disease. There is also a greater spontaneous abortion rate and fetal demise rate among diabetic mothers. Outcome for classes F, H, and R are less positive than the remaining classes.

a. **Symptoms**
For Classes B-T, the expectant mother is diagnosed prior to pregnancy. The symptoms then are related to the level of glucose control as evidenced by objective data, blood glucose levels and glycosylated hemoglobin values obtained at the prenatal visit; and by the maternal subjective symptoms of hypoglycemia or hyperglycemia and her report of self-assessed blood glucose levels. See **Table 1** for symptoms of hypoglycemia and hyperglycemia.

b. **Consequences**
Maternal consequences include increased difficulty of control (tendency toward hypoglycemia in the first trimester and hyperglycemia as pregnancy progresses), hydramnios with the increase in risk for premature rupture of membranes, PIH, ketoacidosis, dystocia, infections (UTI, yeast), and potential progression of vascular involvement.

## Symptoms of Hypoglycemia and Hyperglycemia

| Hypoglycemia | Hyperglycemia |
|---|---|
| Hunger | Thirst |
| Sweating | Nausea |
| Nervous, weak, fatigued | Drowsiness |
| Blurred/double vision | Dim vision |
| Dizziness | Confusion |
| Pale, clammy skin | Flushed, dry skin |
| Shallow respirations | Rapid respirations |
| Normal pulse | Weak, rapid pulse |
|  | Abdominal pain |
|  | Increased urination |
|  | Fruity breath odor |

Embryonic/Fetal/Neonatal consequences include spontaneous abortion, fetal demise, fetal anomaly, intrauterine growth retardation or macrosomia, neonatal hypoglycemia, preterm birth with neonatal respiratory distress syndrome, neonatal hypocalcemia and hypomagnesemia, and neonatal polycythemia and hyperbilirubinemia.

c. **Assessment**
   **Maternal history (risk factors):**

   – Obesity

   – Family history of diabetes mellitus

   – Previous large for gestational age infant(s)

   – Previous hydramnios

   – Previous unexplained fetal demise or stillbirth

   – Previous infant with congenital anomalies

   – Maternal symptoms of diabetes mellitus

   **Maternal well-being:**

   – Lab values (blood glucose, glycosylated hemoglobin)

   – Self-assessed blood glucose

   – Self-report of symptoms

   – Schedule of weight gain

**Fetal well-being:**

- Maternal report of fetal movements

- Fundal height measurements

- MSAFP value

- Non-stress testing results

- Ultrasound evaluation

- Contraction stress testing results

- Other procedures as needed

d. Intervention includes the education provided for nondiabetic expectant mothers plus education regarding dietary management during pregnancy, monitoring blood glucose levels, insulin therapy, balancing exercise with diet and insulin therapy, additional assessment testing (ultrasound, amnio- centesis, NST, CST, biophysical profile), signs and symptoms of complications, and the rationale for more frequent prenatal visits and potential hospital admissions for regulation of insulin therapy. Additional time should be provided at each prenatal visit for the mother to express her feelings and frustrations and even fears regarding the impact of the intensity of control over her life and concern for fetal well-being.

3. **Genitourinary infections that expectant mothers bring to** pregnancy (and that can/do occur in pregnancy) include urinary tract infection (UTI) and sexually transmitted diseases (STDs).

a. UTI symptoms
**Subjective:**

- Backpain

- Dysuria (urgency, frequency, pain)

- Malaise

- Possibly nausea and vomiting

**Objective:**

- Elevated temperature

- Costovertebral angle (CVA) tenderness

- Urinalysis results

- Urine culture results

b. Consequences of UTI include increased risk for maternal pyelonephritis, preterm labor, premature rupture of membranes, and fetal loss.

c. Assessment for UTI includes assessing for subjective and objective symptoms at each prenatal visit. UTI may be present even though the mother is asymptomatic.

d. Intervention for UTI includes reinforcing maternal water intake of 8-10 glasses daily, perineal hygiene measures, reporting of symptoms of dysuria to her primary health care provider, and education for antibiotic therapy. In addition, if routine prenatal "dip stick" urinalysis results are indicative of potential for UTI, a clean catch or catheterized specimen should be evaluated microscopically.

e. STD symptoms are specific to the various STDs. In general, one or more of the following symptoms may occur:

**Subjective:**

- Change in vaginal discharge

  ° Amount

  ° Color

  ° Consistency

  ° Odor

- Perineal itching

- External dysuria

- Dyspareunia

- Presence of lesion(s)

**Objective:**

- Yellowish, greenish, cheese-like, or frothy discharge

- Foul or "fishy" odor of discharge

- Erythematous vaginal and cervical mucosa

- Perineal/vulvar excoriation

- Laboratory test results (wet prep, culture, serum)

f. Consequences of STDs include increased maternal risk for preterm labor, cervical cancer, postpartal endometritis, and/or maternal discomfort. STDs acquired while the woman is not pregnant can increase the risk for pelvic inflammatory disease and resultant infertility problems.

Fetal/neonatal consequences include congenital syphilis (if maternal treatment is omitted or unsuccessful), blindness (ophthalmia neonatorum caused by gonorrhea), conjunctivitis and/or pneumonia (chlamydia), neurological damage or death (herpes type II) and pneumonia or meningitis (group B streptococci).

g. Assessment for STD includes careful history, screening, and follow-up test of cure for the STDs that can be cured.

h. Intervention for STD includes education regarding acquiring, transmitting, preventing, treating, medication instructions, and outcomes of STDs. In addition, education regarding lifestyle risk factors is included in intervention.

4. **Perinatal Human Immunodeficiency Virus (HIV) and Acquired Immunodeficiency Syndrome (AIDS)** is a disorder the mother may bring to pregnancy even though she is unaware that she has been infected. AIDS is diagnosed when a HIV-positive person is diagnosed with any one of the several opportunistic diseases specific to AIDS (such as esophageal candidiasis, herpes simplex virus, wasting syndrome).

Because vulvovaginal candidiasis and cervical dysplasia (common HIV conditions in women) are problems that occur in non-HIV infected women, women tend to initiate HIV treatment at a more advanced stage of the HIV disease than men do. Thus, the expectant mother may not be aware that she is HIV positive when she presents for prenatal care. Further, because of the potential effects of HIV positive status on the fetus/infant, all women should be assessed for HIV exposure. Indeed, failure to offer assessment for HIV infection may be considered to be inappropriate health care. In the future, all states may require HIV screening during pregnancy.

HIV is thought to be transmitted to the fetus/neonate through the following routes: (1) maternal circulation (transplacentally, possibly as early as the first trimester); (2) infected maternal body fluids (during the intrapartal process); and (3) breast milk.

a. **Risk Factors for exposure to HIV include the following:**

   – residing (woman and/or partner) in a HIV infection-prevalent geographic area

   – current or past use of IV drugs (woman and/or partner)

   – current or past exposure to multiple sex partners

   – current or past sex partners who were bisexual or hemophilic

   – blood transfusion(s) between 1978 and 1985

   – current or past occurrence of HIV-related infections

   – personal belief that she has been exposed to HIV

b. Consequences of AIDS include the following:
Maternal Consequences

- Difficulty gaining weight and/or maintaining weight during pregnancy

- Morbidity related to opportunistic diseases

- Passing the disease to others (sexual partner(s), fetus)

- Poor wound healing

- Postpartal endometritis

- Postpartal hemorrhage

- Postpartal UTI

Fetal/Neonatal Consequences

Approximately 50% of neonates that have positive HIV titers will remain HIV positive. [Note: At birth the neonate may have a positive HIV titer because of transfer of maternal HIV antibodies transplacentally. The noninfected infant will lose maternal HIV antibodies by 8-15 months of age. Thus, the infant's own HIV status can be determined by 18 months of age. Most HIV infected infants are asymptomatic at birth but develop symptoms by 3-6 months of age.]

- characteristic facial appearance (if infected, e.g., microcephaly, patulous lips, boxlike prominent forehead, increased distance between inner canthus, flat nasal bridge, mild obliquity of the eyes)

- delayed developmental milestones (if infected)

- mortality (if infected and clinical illness is apparent by 6 months of age, death is common by 12 months of age; average survival from HIV positive test to death is 9 months)

- small for gestational age (if infected)

c. Assessment for Perinatal HIV includes the following:

- assessment for HIV exposure (see above)

- blood testing (Enzyme-Linked ImmunoSorbent Assay to screen for the presence of the HIV antibody; Western Blot Test for diagnosis of HIV infection

- assessment for opportunistic diseases such as the following:

    ° CytoMegalo Virus (CMV)

    ° hepatitis B

- ° mycobacterium tuberculosis
- ° STDs (gonorrhea, syphilis, persistent herpes simplex, candidiasis)
- ° toxoplasmosis
- — assessment for worsening HIV infection includes the folowing:
    - ° chronic diarrhea (lasting longer than one month)
    - ° chronic fever (lasting longer than one month)
    - ° wasting syndrome (weight loss greater than 10% of prepregnant weight)
- d. Interventions for Perinatal HIV includes the following:
    - — Prenatal Period
        - ° zidovudine (ZDV) after 14 weeks gestation to decrease transplacental transmission
        - ° intervention for specific opportunistic diseases
        - ° therapy to prevent/treat anemia
        - ° promotion of expected weight gain
        - ° nutrition counseling
        - ° Trimethoprim prophylaxis for pneumonocystis carinii pneumonia (PCP) if maternal T-cell count is less than 200 cells/cubic millimeter
    - — Intrapartal Period
        - ° usual labor management
        - ° external EFM (to prevent viral inoculation via fetal electrode and/or intrauterine pressure catheter)
        - ° limitation/avoidance of vaginal exams following SROM
        - ° AROM discourged
        - ° standard precautions for blood and body fluids
    - — Neonatal Period
        - ° wipe all fluids from body immediately following birth
        - ° soap and water bath as soon as stable
        - ° delay invasive procedures (heel stick, Vitamin K injection) until bath given
        - ° breast feeding discouraged

- ° ZDV based on CDC recommendations
- ° diapering recommendation (use of disposable diapers, sealing diapers in plastic bags, depositing diapers in garbage cans, frequent diaper changing to avoid skin breakdown; careful handwashing following diaper change; cleansing diaper changing area with 1:10 bleach solution following every diaper change; place diaper changing area away from food handling area)
- ° nutrition to promote weight gain and prevent diarrhea
- ° keeping toys clean and preventing sharing with other children
- ° avoiding rectal temps (stimulate diarrhea)
- ° antimicrobial medications for specific infections for symptomatic neonate
- ° corticosteroids for lymphoid interstitial pneumonitis for symptomatic neonate
- ° prophylaxis for PCP for symptomatic neonate

– Postpartal Period

- ° intervention for postpartal consequences
- ° counseling for maternal care and infant care (treat neonate/infant as HIV positive until infant's HIV status is confirmed)
- ° prevent subsequent pregnancy
- ° referral to provider specializing in HIV/AIDS
- ° referral to support group

# GESTATIONAL DISORDERS

Gestational disorders that occur most often include blood incompatibility, gestational diabetes, hemorrhage, hyperemesis gravidarum, pregnancy-induced hypertension (PIH), and preterm labor. Symptoms, consequences, assessment and intervention for each gestational disorder are summarized below.

1. **Blood incompatibility is due to Rh sensitization of the Rh** negative mother or due to ABO incompatibility. Rh sensitization occurs when the Rh negative mother is exposed to Rh positive red blood cells from a previous pregnancy in which the fetus was Rh positive or a previous Rh positive transfusion.

ABO incompatibility is more common than Rh incompatibility and occurs most often when the mother is type O and the fetus is type A, B, or AB.

The outcome for Rh incompatibility can be a severe disease in the newborn (erythroblastosis fetalis or hydrops fetalis) and intensifies in severity with successive pregnancies in which the fetus is Rh positive. The outcome for ABO incompatibility is usually a much less severe hemolytic disease and severity varies from pregnancy to pregnancy.

The pathology of blood incompatibility is the passage of the anti-Rh positive or anti-A/anti-B antibodies from the mother across the placenta to the fetus where the antibodies cause hemolysis of fetal red blood cells.

a. Symptoms do not occur in the mother. Neonatal symptoms are:

   – Hyperbilirubinemia

   – Anemia

   – Edema (untreated Rh incompatibility)

b. Consequences for the fetus/neonate include anemia, hyperbilirubinemia, fetal demise (severe Rh incompatibility) and risk for neonatal kernicterus.

c. Assessment includes assessment of maternal Rh factor and Rh sensitization (indirect Coomb's) during pregnancy. If Rh sensitization has occurred, additional assessment procedures such as amniocentesis and ultrasound may be performed. Assessment for ABO incompatibility occurs after birth of the neonate and includes blood type and Rh, hemoglobin and hematocrit, and bilirubin levels. The same neonatal laboratory assessments occur in the neonate with an Rh incompatibility.

d. Intervention includes education regarding assessment tests, treatment procedures, and outcomes and counseling regarding emotional support by significant others.

2. **Gestational diabetes is diabetes mellitus that is glucose** intolerance that is first diagnosed during pregnancy and is caused by the diabetogenic effect of pregnancy. The elevated levels of the pregnancy hormones (especially human placental lactogen, estrogen, progesterone, and cortisol) decrease the effectiveness of insulin. The body responds by increasing the production of insulin as pregnancy progresses. If the maternal pancreas is unable to increase the insulin production sufficiently to overcome the effects of the hormones, hyperglycemia (diabetes mellitus) results. Thus, gestational diabetes mellitus (GDM) is classified in White's classification as Class A diabetes mellitus.

The outcome for GDM can be approximately the same as for a pregnancy that is not complicated by GDM, if glycemic control is maintained. Often, the outcome is a large-for-gestational-age (macrosomic) neonate.

   **a.** Symptoms may include the typical symptoms of polyuria, polydipsia, weight loss, and polyphagia. However, the expectant mother may experience increased weight gain, thirst, and glycosuria.

   **b.** Consequences for the mother include distress due to the diagnosis, change in life-style, and concern for fetal well-being. In addition, she is at greater risk for genitourinary infection, dystocia, and cesarean birth, as well as complications due to diabetes mellitus above (PIH, hydramnios, ketoacidosis).

   Fetal consequences include the consequences identified above for the fetus/neonate (macrosomia, hypoglycemia, hyperbilirubinemia, respiratory distress syndrome, hypocalcemia).

   **c.** Assessment begins with the initial maternal history for risk factors, includes urine testing for glucose and ketones at each prenatal visit, and early glucose screening for mothers with positive history of risk factors or symptoms, plus the usually-scheduled glucose screen at 24-28 weeks.

   **d.** Intervention includes counseling regarding the new diagnosis of GDM and the educational interventions similar to those for the expectant mother who was diagnosed with diabetes mellitus prior to pregnancy, including learning to perform blood glucose assessments and administration of insulin.

**3. Hemorrhage can be divided roughly into occurrences early** In pregnancy and occurrences in latter pregnancy. Early pregnancy hemorrhage is due to one of the types of abortion, ectopic pregnancy, or due to the presence of hydatidiform mole. Hemorrhage in the latter part of pregnancy is usually caused by abruptio placentae or placenta previa.

   **a.** Symptoms of early pregnancy hemorrhage include the following:

      – Some bleeding, mild cramping or backache, and closed cervical os (threatened abortion)

      – Moderate bleeding, moderate cramping, open cervical os (inevitable abortion or imminent abortion))

      – Heavy bleeding, severe cramping, open cervical os, passage of tissue (incomplete abortion)

- Passage of tissue followed by slight bleeding, mild cramping, closed cervical os, uterine size small for dates (complete abortion)

- Slight dark bleeding or discharge, no cramping, closed cervical os, no passage of tissue, uterine size small for dates (missed abortion)

- Relatively bloodless, relatively painless, open cervical os, passage of tissue (Repetitive second trimester abortions due to cervical incompetency or dysfunction)

- Missed menstrual period, slight bleeding, adnexal fullness, unilateral pelvic pain, possible shock out of proportion to amount of observable bleeding and possible referred shoulder pain (ruptured ectopic pregnancy)

- Scant to profuse dark or bright red bleeding, abdominal cramping, usually uterine size greater than dates but may have uterine size smaller than dates, absence of FHR, excessive nausea and vomiting, and possible development of PIH before 20 weeks (hydatidiform mole)

b. Consequences of early pregnancy hemorrhage include fetal loss, potential for hemorrhage, parental grieving or loss of a fallopian tube with ectopic pregnancy or risk for uterine rupture or development of choriocarcinoma with hydatidiform mole.

c. Assessment of early pregnancy hemorrhage includes subjective and objective symptoms, history of LMP, and maternal/paternal feelings and support systems.

d. Intervention for early pregnancy hemorrhage includeseducation regarding assessment and treatment procedures, discharge, follow-up procedures, life-style habits that may be related to pregnancy loss, and referral for grief counseling. In addition, listening to the parents talk about the pregnancy, and the loss as a means of supporting them is supportive therapy.

e. Symptoms of latter pregnancy hemorrhage are due to abruptio placentae (premature separation of a normally implanted placenta) or placenta previa (abnormal implantation of the placenta in the lower uterine segment near or over the cervical os) and include these symptoms:

## Symptoms of Abruptio Placentae and Placenta Previa

| Abruptio Placentae | Placenta Previa |
|---|---|
| Absent to severe pain | No pain |
| Concealed or obvious bleeding | Small to heavy bleeding |
| Dark red blood if obvious | Bright red blood |
| Bleeding continuous if obvious | Bleeding intermittent |
| Uterine tone normal to boardlike | Normal uterine tone |
| Fetal position normal | Fetal position abnormal |
| Increase in fundal height due to bleeding | No increase in fundal height due to bleeding |
| Shock absent to severe | Shock (occasional) |
| PIH common | PIH not usual |
| Coagulopathy occasional to common | Coagulopathy rare |
| History of trauma, hypertension, or cocaine use and previous abruptio placentae | |

f. **Consequences:**
Consequences of abruptio placentae include potential for maternal disseminated intravascular coagulopathy (DIC), maternal and fetal mortality, and risk for neonatal neurological damage.

Consequences of placenta previa include risk for maternal postpartal hemorrhage (implantation site is passive portion of uterus), cesarean birth, anemia, and infection.

g. **Assessment:**
Assessment of abruptio placentae includes symptoms, vital signs, DIC, fetal viability/well-being, laboratory tests (including coagulation testing), increase in fundal height (indication of concealed bleeding), maternal and paternal anxiety level. Symptoms of DIC include purpura, bleeding from mucous membranes, GI bleeding, or bleeding from any orifice.

Assessment of placenta previa includes symptoms, vital signs, fetal well-being, laboratory tests, and maternal/paternal anxiety level. In addition, prenatal assessment of abnormal fetal position and placental souffle in the lower uterine segment are indications for further assessment procedures (ultrasound) to rule out placenta previa.

h. **Intervention:**
Intervention for abruptio placentae includes education regarding definition of abruptio placentae, potential causes, assessment and treatment procedures, potential outcomes, potential for cesarean birth, recovery, discharge, and follow-up, as well as parental emotional support during the crisis.

Intervention for placenta previa includes education regarding definition of placenta previa, consequences, potential cause, bed rest and hospitalizations, assessment and treatment procedures, potential outcomes, potential for cesarean birth, recovery, discharge, and follow-up, as well as maternal emotional support during hospitalizations and prenatal visits.

4. **Hyperemesis gravidarum is excessive or exaggerated** nausea and vomiting of pregnancy that results in electrolyte, nutritional, and metabolic imbalances. The cause may be elevated estrogen levels and the higher HCG levels of the first trimester, especially increased with multiple gestation and hydatidiform mole. With restoration of the imbalances and completion of the first trimester, the outcome is essentially the same as for pregnancies not complicated by hyperemesis gravidarum. If the imbalances are not corrected, intrauterine growth retardation, CNS malforma- tions, and embryonic/fetal death may be the outcome for the neonate.

a. **Symptoms:**
   - Vomiting of all intake

   - Retching between oral intake

   - Dehydration

   - Fluid and electrolyte imbalances

   - Hypotension

   - Tachycardia

   - Increased hematocrit and BUN

   - Oliguria

   - Metabolic acidosis

   - Weight loss

   - Jaundice

   - Starvation

b. Consequences for the mother include the imbalances and symptoms listed above. If the imbalances cannot be corrected the pregnancy may need to be interrupted to preserve the health and life of the mother. Consequences for the fetus may

be fetal death for uncorrected, severe hyperemesis gravidarum.

c. Assessment includes history, symptoms, laboratory tests, and
embryo/fetal well-being.

d. Intervention includes education regarding the disorder,
symptoms, assessment and treatment procedures, and
outcomes, accurate I&O (including emesis), oral hygiene, and
maternal emotional support.

5. **PIH (Pregnancy-Induced Hypertension) is characterized by**
hypertension, proteinuria, and edema. PIH is classified as mild or
severe preeclampsia based on severity of symptoms. It is classified as eclampsia once convulsions occur, or as HELLP (Hemolysis, Elevated Liver enzymes, and Low Platelet count) Syndrome
when preeclampsia and eclampsia have increased in severity.

The cause is unknown but the resulting pathophysiology involves
arterial vasospasm which causes decreased organ perfusion, and
the symptoms of the disorder. It is cured by termination of the
pregnancy and occurs before 20 weeks gestation in the presence
of hydatidiform mole. It seems to occur in families, first pregnancies, mothers with inadequate nutrition (especially low protein
intake), teen mothers, mothers over 35 years of age, and low
socioeconomic mothers.

Outcome is dependent upon the severity and duration of the
disorder. Vasospasm and resultant decreased organ perfusion
(especially the placenta) results in intrauterine growth retardation
for the fetus. Maternal hospitalization for assessment and intervention is often required. Early birth is often required for severe
PIH.

a. Symptoms are based on severity of the disorder as follows:
**Mild preeclampsia:**

– Hypertension (increase of 30/15 mm Hg or more)

– Proteinuria (1+ to 2+ by dipstick)

– Edema (dependent plus puffiness of fingers and face)

– Weight gain (>1 lb/week)

**Severe preeclampsia:**

– Hypertension (160/110 mm Hg or more)

– Proteinuria (2+ or greater by dip stick)

– Edema (generalized, pulmonary edema)

– Hyperreflexia

– Weight gain (>1 lb/week; may be sudden increase)

- Oliguria

- Severe headache

- Visual disturbances (blurred, photophobia, spots)

- Severe irritability

- Epigastric pain and/or nausea and vomiting

- Elevated serum creatinine

- Thrombocytopenia

- AST markedly elevated

- Increased hematocrit (hemoconcentration)

**Eclampsia:**

- Symptoms of severe preeclampsia

- Convulsions

**HELLP syndrome:**

- Symptoms of severe preeclampsia

- Hemolysis

- AST and ALT elevated

- Platelet count (low)

- BUN and creatinine elevated

- Creatinine elevated

b. Consequences:
Maternal consequences include increased morbidity and mortality, increased risk for abruptio placentae and DIC, and increased risk for cerebral hemorrhage, hepatic failure, and acute renal failure.

Fetal consequences include intrauterine growth retardation, increased risk for fetal demise, and increased risk for neonatal mortality and morbidity.

c. Assessment includes monitoring for presence and increased severity of symptoms, laboratory tests, fetal well-being, symptoms of abruptio placentae, symptoms of DIC, maternal anxiety level, and maternal support systems.

d. Intervention includes convulsion precautions; education of mother and family regarding disorder process, consequences, potential outcomes, assessment and treatment procedures, coping measures for complete bed rest, stress reduction measures, preparation for birth, recovery, discharge, and follow-up; and administration of medications.

Medications commonly administered include Magnesium Sulfate (antidote is Calcium Gluconate), fluid and electrolyte replacement, Valium or phenobarbital as sedatives, and Apresoline (antihypertensive).

6. **Preterm labor is defined as labor that occurs after 20 weeks** gestation and before completion of 37 weeks of gestation. The exact cause is not known but preterm labor has occurred following premature rupture of membranes, UTI, chorioam- nionitis, abruptio placentae, incompetent cervix, and with multiple (fetal) gestation, cardiovascular or renal disease, diabetes mellitus, PIH, chlamydial vaginitis, maternal smoking more than one pack per day, low socioeconomic status, hydramnios, age less than 17 or greater than 34 years, and previous preterm births.

   The outcome is dependent on gestational age of the fetus at the time of birth. The preterm neonate is at risk for morbidity and mortality because of the immaturity of organs and systems.

   a. **Symptoms** include rupture of membranes, intermittent backache, pelvic pressure, sudden increase in vaginal discharge, and/or 6 or more uterine contractions of at least 30 seconds duration in one hour.

   b. **Consequences**:
      Maternal consequences include anxiety regarding the well-being of the fetus/neonate and the impact of medications used to delay birth.

      Fetal consequences include increased risk for morbidity and mortality associated with immature organs and systems with preterm birth, especially the immature respiratory system.

   c. Assessment includes monitoring for symptoms of labor, fetal well-being, and effect of tocolytic therapy on mother and fetus.

   d. Interventions include anxiety/stress reduction measures for the mother, administration and monitoring of medications, education regarding assessment and treatment procedures, potential cause of preterm labor, outcome, preparation for inevitable labor, recovery, care of the neonate, discharge, and follow-up.

      Medications administered as tocolytics include Magnesium Sulfate, Terbutaline, and Yutopar. In addition, glucocorticoids may be administered to enhance fetal lung maturity.

# *Unit 2*

## THE INTRAPARTAL PERIOD

*The intrapartal period is that portion of the childbearing process that involves labor, birth, and postdelivery recovery. The unit focuses on the birthing process; maternal, fetal, and neonatal assessment; nursing interventions; and selected intrapartal complications.*

CHAPTER 7

# THE PROCESS OF BIRTH

*The process of birth consists of four stages of labor involving enormous maternal work to accomplish dilatation of the cervix, expulsion of the fetus from the uterus, and passage of the placenta. Initiation of labor, signs of labor, the critical components of the process, the mechanisms of labor, and the stages of labor are essential concepts in understanding the birthing process.*

## THE INITIATION OF LABOR

The cause of the onset of labor has not been clearly determined. Several theories have been proposed to explain the cause of labor. A summary of the major theories follows:

1. The **stretch theory** postulates that when the uterus has stretched to full capacity, labor begins and the uterus is emptied.

2. The **oxytocin theory** postulates that the posterior pituitary releases oxytocin at term to initiate labor. The uterus does become more responsive to oxytocin stimulation as term approaches. Oxytocin is administered to induce labor.

3. The **progesterone withdrawal theory** postulates that the level of progesterone decreases at term, allowing uterine contractions to occur. The change in progesterone level may permit prostaglandin production which in turn stimulates uterine contractions.

4. The **estrogen stimulation theory** postulates that estrogen irritates the uterine myometrium and may facilitate production of prostaglandin.

5. The **fetal cortisol theory** postulates that the fetal cortisol may play a role in prostaglandin production and in decreased progesterone levels.

6. The **fetal membrane phospholipid-arachidonic acid-prostaglandin theory** postulates that prostaglandin may stimulate oxytocin production. Prostaglandin does stimulate uterine contractions and production does increase immediately prior to labor.

## SIGNS OF LABOR

The signs of labor can be classified into the premonitory signs, false labor signs, and true labor signs. The expectant mother may confuse the premonitory and false labor signs with true labor. True labor is determined by physical assessment of the cervix to evaluate the ability of the observed signs to cause cervical change.

## Premonitory Signs of Labor

**Premonitory signs of labor** are those signs that occur several hours to several days before the onset of labor. They serve as an advanced warning or "premonition" that labor is impending. The expectant mother may notice one or more of the signs. The signs include:

1. **Lightening** is the beginning of descent of the fetus into the pelvis. It occurs in primigravid mothers 2-3 weeks before the onset of labor and may not occur in multiparous mothers until sometime in the labor process.

2. **Braxton-Hicks contractions** are the irregular, intermittent, mild uterine contractions that have been occurring throughout pregnancy but were undetected by the expectant mother until near term. They become increasingly stronger until they cause maternal discomfort and are frequently confused as the begin- ning of labor. Because they do not produce progressive change in the cervix, they are termed "false labor contractions."

3. **Cervical changes** such as becoming softer, initial effacement, and initial dilatation begin to occur a few days before the onset of labor.

4. **Bloody show** occurs with passage of the mucous plug, consists of a small amount of blood mixed with mucus, and is pinkish in color. This sign usually occurs a few hours before the onset of labor.

5. **Burst of energy** occurs a few hours before the onset of labor. The mother suddenly feels very energetic and may be motivated to complete house cleaning, baking, and other activities previously omitted because of feelings of fatigue. The energy should be saved for labor.

6. **Spontaneous rupture of membranes** is revealed as a sudden gush of fluid escaping from the vagina and cannot be controlled by the mother. It can occur 12-24 hours before the onset of labor, or it may not occur until labor is well established.

## False Labor Signs

**False labor signs** are characteristics of uterine contractions that the expectant mother notices. However, the false labor contractions do not cause a progressive change in the cervix. The characteristics include the following:

1. The **frequency** of the false labor uterine contractions is irregular.

   The **frequency of uterine contractions** is how often the contractions are occurring and is determined by counting the time from the beginning of one contraction to the beginning of the next contraction for several contractions.

2. The **duration** of the false labor uterine contractions is variable but is seldom greater than 30 seconds.

   The **duration of uterine contractions** is how long the contractions last and is determined by counting the time from the beginning of the contraction to the end of the contraction.

3. The **intensity** of false labor uterine contractions usually remains about the same.

   The **intensity of uterine contractions** is how strong they are and is determined by palpation or by intrauterine catheter pressure readings.

4. The **location of discomfort** of false labor uterine contractions is primarily felt in the abdomen.

5. A **change in activity** may cause false labor uterine contractions to cease.

6. The **cervix** does not change as a result of false labor uterine contractions.

## True Labor Signs

The **true labor signs** are characteristics of uterine contractions noticed by the expectant mother and when assessed by a health care provider are determined to cause progressive change (effacement and dilatation) in the cervix. The characteristics include the following:

1. The **frequency** of the uterine contractions is regular and the resting time between them becomes progressively shorter.

   **Resting time** is determined by counting the time from the end of one contraction to the beginning of the next contraction.

2. The **duration** of the uterine contractions progressively increases.

3. The **intensity** of the uterine contractions progressively increases.

4. The **location** of the discomfort of the uterine contractions is first felt in the back and then in the abdomen.

5. A **change in activity** may intensify the discomfort of the uterine contractions (walking) or have no effect (lying down).

6. The **cervix** does show progressive change in effacement and dilatation as a result of the uterine contractions.

# CRITICAL COMPONENTS OF THE PROCESS

The **critical components** of the birthing process determine the progress and outcome. The components include the passage, passenger, power, placenta, maternal and fetal physiological response to labor, and the maternal psychological response to labor. Each component is summarized below:

1. The **passage** is the path the fetus negotiates in order to pass from the uterus to the extrauterine environment. It consists of the maternal pelvis and the cervical, vaginal, and perineal soft tissues.

   a. The **bony pelvis** is divided into the false pelvis (the portion above the brim or pelvic inlet) and the true pelvis (the portion below the brim). The true pelvis consists of the inlet, mid-pelvis, and outlet. The diameters of the inlet, mid-pelvis, and outlet determine the type of pelvis and whether or not the fetus will be able to pass through the pelvis.

   b. The four primary **types of pelvis** are the gynecoid (female), android (male), anthropoid (ape-like), and platypelloid (flat). The gynecoid pelvis is the type with pelvic diameters and features that are most favorable to vaginal birth. Relaxin permits an increase in pelvic diameters by relaxing the pelvic joints, especially the symphysis pubis.

   c. There are several **pelvic diameters** that can be determined for the inlet, mid-pelvis, and outlet.

   The **obstetric conjugate** is the inlet diameter that determines whether or not the fetal presenting part can engage. Since the obstetric conjugate cannot be determined directly on physical exam it is estimated by subtracting 1.5- 2.0 cm from the diagonal conjugate (which should measure 12.5-13 cm in the gynecoid pelvis).

   The **interspinous diameter** (10.5 cm) is the smallest diameter of the mid-pelvis and determines whether or not the presenting part can pass through the mid-pelvis.

   An important outlet diameter is the **transverse diameter** of the outlet (10-11 cm).

2. The **passenger** is the fetus. The determinants of the movement of the passenger through the passage include the size of the fetal head, the fetal presentation, the fetal position, the fetal lie, and the fetal attitude.

   a. The **size of the fetal head** is based on the diameters of the fetal skull and the amount of molding (the overlapping of the bones of the skull) that occurs during labor.

The diameters of the fetal skull need to fit with the maternal pelvic diameters as the fetal head descends into and through the maternal pelvis. Fetal position determines which fetal skull diameters present in the maternal pelvic inlet, mid-pelvis and outlet.

Molding is permitted because of the connection of the bones of the fetal skull by sutures (fibrous membrane connections) and the fetal skull fontanelles ("soft" spot at the junction of the skull bones). The membranous connections and fontanelles permit the skull bones to overlap each other during passage through the birth canal.

b. The **fetal presentation** is determined by the fetal body part (the presenting part) that enters the maternal pelvis first. The most common fetal presentation is cephalic (head) with breech presentation (buttocks) being next common. Other fetal presentations, such as shoulder, are considered abnormal presentations.

c. The **fetal position** is the relationship of the landmark on the fetal presenting part to the quadrants of the maternal pelvis (left anterior, right anterior, left posterior, right posterior). The position is recorded by using the first letter for the right or left side of the maternal pelvis, the first letter of the fetal presenting part landmark, and the first letter for the anterior or posterior portion of the maternal pelvis.

For example, the occiput is the most common presenting part of the fetal skull. If the occiput is located in the left anterior quadrant of the maternal pelvis, the fetal position is recorded as left occiput anterior or LOA where "L" stands for the left side of the maternal pelvis, "O" stands for the fetal presenting part landmark, the occiput, and "A" stands for the anterior portion of the maternal pelvis.

The usual fetal presenting part landmark for breech presentation is the sacrum, for shoulder presentation is the acromion process or shoulder, and for face presentation is the mentum (chin).

d. The **fetal lie** is the relationship of the fetal spine (long axis or cephalocaudal axis) to the maternal spine. The usual lie is longitudinal (the two axes are parallel). With longitudinal or vertical lie, the presentation would be cephalic or breech. The unusual lie is the transverse (horizontal) lie where the two axes are perpendicular. With the transverse lie, the presentation is usually a shoulder presentation.

e. The **fetal attitude** is the relationship of the body parts of fetus to each other. The usual attitude is one of flexion, where the head is flexed with the chin resting on the chest, the arms flexed on the chest, and the legs flexed on the abdomen.

3. The **power** is the rhythmic, "automatic" contractions of the uterine myometrium that accomplish cervical dilatation and effacement, and descent of the fetus in the maternal pelvis. The uterine contractions occur in a wave-like pattern beginning in the fundus and pushing the fetal presenting part against the cervix and at the same time pulling the cervix up around the fetal presenting part to accomplish cervical dilatation and effacement. The uterine contractions are described by their frequency, duration, and intensity.

   Once cervical dilation and effacement are completed, the additional power of voluntary maternal abdominal muscle contractions are added to the primary power of the uterine contractions to help push the fetus through the birth canal.

4. The **placenta** is a critical component of labor because of its location, attachment, and ability to support the fetus during the birthing process. The placenta previa determines outcome because of its location, abruptio placentae impacts outcome because of its premature separation, and placental insufficiency places the fetus at risk for intrauterine hypoxia and anoxia. Thus, the normally implanted placenta in the upper uterine segment that functions sufficiently to prevent fetal hypoxia facilitates achieving a positive neonatal outcome.

5. The maternal **physiological response** involves the cardiovascular, respiratory, gastrointestinal, renal, integumentary, endocrine, musculoskeletal, and neurologic system changes.

   a. The **cardiovascular system changes** that take place during uterine contractions include increased cardiac output, increased blood pressure, and decreased pulse. During labor, increased WBC occurs. The cause for the increased WBC is thought to be caused by the stress of labor. The primary cause for the other changes is due to redistribution of blood flow during uterine contractions. In addition, the use of the valsalva maneuver during pushing causes an increase in intrathoracic pressure and resulting increase in venous pressure. Maternal supine position intensifies the risk for the occurrence of hypotension.

   b. The **respiratory system changes** include increased oxygen consumption and respiratory rate. In addition, anxiety may result in hyperventilation with resulting respiratory alkalosis. The cause of increased oxygen consumption is due to uterine contractions.

   c. The **gastrointestinal system changes** include decreased motility, decreased absorption, and increased stomach emptying time due to shift in blood flow away from the GI system and due to pressure from the contracting uterus. In addition, nausea and vomiting of undigested food is not unusual, and diarrhea may occur with labor.

d. The **renal system changes** include diaphoresis, increased insensible water loss, difficulty emptying the bladder, and potential for proteinuria. Thirst and temperature elevation may occur due to diaphoresis and insensible water loss precipitated by the work of labor and increased respirations (especially with hyperventilation). Pressure from descent of the fetus can result in tissue edema and inability to void. A full bladder is palpable and visible above the symphysis. Protein in the urine occurs in response to muscle tissue breakdown secondary to the increased physical work of labor.

e. The **integumentary system changes** include the distensibility of the perineum and vaginal introitus. The vaginal introitus must dilate 10 cm (just as the cervix) in order for birth to occur. Lacerations may occur.

f. The **endocrine system changes** include a decrease in progesterone production; an increase in estrogen, prostaglandin, and oxytocin production; and a decrease in maternal glucose level in response to the increase in metabolism prompted by the increased physical work of labor.

g. The **musculoskeletal system changes** include the effects of relaxin (increased relaxation of joints), diaphoresis, fatigue, and leg cramps.

h. The **neurologic system changes** include those precipitated by the discomfort and stress of labor. Pain during the dilatation and effacement portion of labor (first stage) is caused by cervical dilatation, myometrium hypoxia during uterine contractions, stretching of the lower uterine segment, and pressure on lower abdominal and pelvic tissue. Because the contractions are intermittent, maternal discomfort is perceived during contractions and relief is experienced between contractions.

Pain during the second stage of labor is due to myometrial hypoxia, vaginal and perineal distention, and soft tissue pressure. The perineal discomfort is more of a burning than a pain sensation.

Fatigue and sleep deprivation intensify the perception of discomfort and decrease the coping capability of the mother.

6. The **fetal physiological response to the birthing process** includes cardiovascular system, respiratory system, neurologic system, integumentary system, and musculoskeletal system changes or responses.

a. **Cardiovascular system** changes include fetal heart rate responses to constriction of uterine vessels and reduced oxygenation during uterine contractions and changes in fetal circulation in response to maternal position, uterine contractions, maternal blood pressure, and umbilical cord blood flow.

b. **Respiratory system** changes include fetal respiratory movements, fetal body movements, and the facilitation of neonatal respiration by the removal of a portion of the amniotic fluid from the lungs by the pressure exerted on the chest as the fetus moves through the birth canal in a vaginal birth.

c. **Neurologic system** changes include the decrease in fetal heart rate in response to pressure exerted on the fetal head and the characteristic changes in the fetal heart rate pattern in response to stimulation of the fetal sympathetic and parasympathetic divisions of the autonomic nervous system during the birthing process. Stimulation of the sympathetic division increases the fetal heart rate. Stimulation of the parasympathetic division decreases the heart rate and maintains the short-term variability of the heart rate pattern.

d. **Integumentary system** changes occur because of pressure on fetal body parts during the process. Observable changes include the occurrence of caput succedaneum, cephalohematoma, and petechiae or ecchymosis.

e. **Musculoskeletal system** changes include the attitude assumed by the fetus because of the pressure exerted by the contracting uterus and the passage through the birth canal.

7. The maternal **psychological response** is primarily the response to the discomfort of labor. It depends on the mother's preparation for the experience, past experiences with pain, learned cultural responses, fatigue level, and fear/anxiety level.

The psychological response can also be categorized according to stage and phase of labor. During early labor (latent phase), the mother tends to be excited that labor is finally beginning, confident that she can cope with the discomfort, talkative, and eager to see her neonate. During the active phase, the mother is more uncomfortable, begins to doubt her ability to cope, becomes more introverted, and experiences more anxiety. During the transition phase, the mother is extremely uncomfortable, very introverted, convinced that she cannot cope with the discomfort, irritable, indecisive, restless, fearful, fatigued, and very anxious. During the second stage, the mother is relieved that the contractions do not appear as painful and that the birth seems to be near. She usually becomes excited about the impending birth and works to cooperate with her pushing efforts to hasten the birth. If the second stage is prolonged, the mother may become very fatigued and irritable. During the third stage, the mother is very excited about the baby and relieved that labor is over. During the fourth stage, the mother is tired, sleepy, hungry, and thirsty.

# MECHANISMS OF LABOR

The **mechanisms of labor** are the cardinal movements or changes in attitude and position that the fetus assumes to adjust to the maternal pelvis during the passage through the birth canal. The changes must occur in order and include engagement, descent, flexion, internal rotation, extension, restitution, external rotation, and expulsion.

1. **Engagement** is the beginning of descent and occurs when the fetal head biparietal diameter has passed the maternal pelvic inlet. Ideally, the position of the fetal head at engagement is LOT or ROT (left or right occiput transverse) in order to accommodate to the widest diameter (transverse diameter) of the maternal pelvic inlet of the gynecoid pelvis.

2. **Descent** is the progressive movement of the fetus through the maternal pelvis. Descent is more rapid during the latter part of the first stage of labor and during the second stage.

   Descent is determined by assessing the location of the fetal presenting part in relation to the maternal pelvic ischial spines (the station) and designating the location by the number of centimeters the presenting part is above or below the level of the ischial spines. If the fetal presenting part is above the level of the ischial spines, the station is recorded as a negative value. If the presenting part is below the level of the ischial spines, the station is recorded as a positive value. For example, the station of a presenting part that is two centimeters above the level of the ischial spines would be recorded as a -2 station. If the presenting part is at the level of the ischial spines, the station is recorded as zero.

3. **Flexion** is a further flexion of the fetal head with the fetal chin resting on the fetal chest. This maneuver permits the smaller fetal head diameter, the suboccipitobregmatic diameter, to present to the maternal outlet. Flexion occurs when the fetal presenting part pushes against the cervix and pelvic floor musculature.

4. **Internal rotation** is a change in position of the fetal head to accommodate the widest diameter of the maternal mid-pelvis and outlet which is the anterior-posterior diameter. The fetal head position rotates to an occiput anterior position. The position change occurs due to resistance from the bony pelvis and the musculature of the maternal pelvic floor.

5. **Extension** is the pivoting motion of the fetal occiput as it passes under the maternal symphysis as the fetal head is born.

6. **Restitution** is the rotation of the fetal head after it has passed through the introitus so that it can align with the fetal shoulders which have entered the maternal pelvic inlet in the transverse position to accommodate to the widest diameter (following the same path as the fetal head).

7. **External rotation** is further rotation of the fetal head to align again with the fetal shoulders as the shoulders reach the maternal mid-pelvis and rotate to an anterior-posterior position to accommodate the mid-pelvic and pelvic outlet anterior-posterior diameters. The anterior shoulder then rotates under the maternal pelvic symphysis and is born first, followed quickly by birth of the posterior shoulder.

8. **Expulsion** is the rapid birth of the body of the fetus that occurs following birth of the head and shoulders.

## STAGES OF LABOR

The four stages of labor are termed the first, second, third, and fourth stages of labor. The stages are defined as follows:

1. The **first stage of labor** begins with the onset of regular uterine contractions and ends with complete dilatation of the cervix (10 cm). It consists of three phases, the latent phase, active phase, and transition phase.

   a. The **latent phase** is from the onset of regular uterine contractions to cervical dilatation of 3-4 cm. It is the longest phase of the first stage and averages about 8.5 hours for the primigravida and 5 hours for the multipara. Cervical effacement and dilatation occur with little fetal presenting part descent. Uterine contractions are mild with a beginning frequency of 10-20 minutes and a duration of 15-30 seconds and finally develop a frequency of 5-7 minutes and a duration of 30-40 seconds with an increase in intensity.

   b. The **active phase** lasts from the time cervical dilatation is 4 cm until it reaches 8 cm. The uterine contractions at the beginning of the active phase are moderate in tone with a frequency of 2-3 minutes and duration of 60 seconds. The intensity of the contractions increases during the active phase to strong with the continued frequency of 2-3 minutes and duration of 60 seconds. Descent of the fetal presenting part begins during this phase and cervical change continues.

   c. The **transition phase** is the shortest and most painful phase of the first stage. It lasts from the time of 8 cm cervical dilatation to 10 cm dilatation. The fetal presenting part descends more rapidly during the transition phase. Uterine contraction frequency is 1.5-2 minutes, duration is 60-90 seconds and tone/intensity is strong.

2. The **second stage of labor** is from complete dilatation of the cervix until birth of the fetus. It averages approximately 1 hour in primigravid mothers and 15 minutes in multiparous mothers. Rapid descent of the fetal presenting part is accomplished. Uterine contraction frequency may slow slightly at the beginning of the second stage and then return to a frequency of 1.5-2 minutes and a duration of 60-90 seconds with a strong intensity. Maternal bearing down/pushing efforts facilitate birth of the fetus.

3. The **third stage of labor** is the period of time from birth of the fetus to delivery of the placenta. It averages 5-15 minutes.

4. The **fourth stage of labor** is the immediate postdelivery recovery period beginning following delivery of the placenta and lasting 1-4 hours.

# CHAPTER 8

# MATERNAL, FETAL, AND NEONATAL ASSESSMENT

*Intrapartal assessment involves review of the prenatal record and recording of a thorough pregnancy history, admission physical assessment, ongoing maternal and fetal well-being assessment, and the immediate post-delivery assessment of the neonate. Changes in maternal and/or fetal status can occur quickly. Thus, frequent or continuous assessment is necessary and requires use of all nursing assessment skills, such as palpation, auscultation, listening, and careful observation.*

## PRENATAL RECORD REVIEW AND PREGNANCY HISTORY

### Prenatal Record Review

**The review of the prenatal record** provides relevant data regarding past and current medical history of the expectant mother, her family, and her partner; obstetric and gynecologic history; occupational history; and social, cultural, and developmental history. In addition, it provides data regarding personal risk factors, life-style risk factors, past history risk factors, initial physical assessment, and current pregnancy history and risk factors. The data from the prenatal record need to be evaluated for potential impact on labor progress and outcome.

### Pregnancy History

The **current pregnancy history** includes data from the prenatal record, a history of the current labor process from the onset to arrival at the birthing facility, and any changes in prenatal record data the mother desires regarding choice of analgesic/anesthesia, infant feeding, and pediatrician. Planned methods for coping with the discomfort of labor, expectations for the birthing process, agreements made with her primary health provider, and effectiveness of coping measures used so far should be reviewed by the admitting nurse.

## ADMISSION PHYSICAL ASSESSMENT

The **admission physical assessment** focuses on determining the maternal physical and psychologic well-being, labor status, and fetal well-being. It is not as thorough as the initial prenatal assessment but is essential for determining maternal and fetal status.

**1. Maternal physical well-being assessment** includes vital signs, heart and lung sounds, weight gain, fundal height, edema, and laboratory test assessment. A summary of each component follows:

a. **Vital signs** include maternal blood pressure, temperature, pulse, and respirations. Maternal blood pressure is assessed between uterine contractions to establish an accurate baseline value because of the tendency of the blood pressure to rise during uterine contractions. The blood pressure value is compared with the baseline value obtained in early pregnancy as recorded in the prenatal record in order to evaluate the potential for occurrence of PIH during labor or the occurrence of supine hypotension.

Maternal temperature is evaluated for potential development of intrapartal uterine infection (especially with rupture of membranes) or for maternal dehydration.

Tachycardia and tachypnea may indicate cardiac and respiratory disorders or maternal anxiety.

b. **Heart sounds** are assessed for the presence of murmurs. If a murmur is detected, it must be evaluated to determine the cause (cardiac disease or pregnancy induced due to extra blood volume and cardiac output).

c. **Lung sounds** are auscultated for occurrence of abnormal sounds indicating the potential for infection.

d. **Weight gain** total for pregnancy is evaluated for anticipation of the birth of a large or small for gestational age neonate or the potential for PIH (generalized edema).

e. **Fundal height** provides data for evaluating fetal size for gestational age, occurrence of hydramnios or oligohy- dramnios, prematurity, or multiple gestation.

f. **Edema** is evaluated to differentiate between the expected dependent edema of pregnancy and generalized edema which would indicate the potential for development of PIH during labor.

If generalized edema is present, deep tendon reflexes would also be assessed for further signs of PIH.

g. **Laboratory test assessment** includes a CBC, serology, and urinalysis. The CBC provides data regarding infection or anemia. The serology identifies the presence of syphilis. If the serology is positive for syphilis, neonatal treatment and planning for care should be anticipated. The urine is evalu-ated for presence of ketones, protein, RBCs and WBCs. Ketones and glucose in the urine indicate the need to assess serum glucose levels. Proteinuria indicates the need to assess for

PIH or UTI. RBCs and WBCs indicate the need to assess for UTI.

2. **Labor status** includes assessment of uterine contractions, cervix, station, and membranes. A summary of each component follows:

   a. **Uterine contractions** are assessed for frequency, duration, intensity, resting time, and resting tone. See Intrapartal Chapter 1 for definition of frequency, duration and resting time. **Note:** Oxygen, nutrient, and waste exchange requires at least 30 seconds resting time between contractions.

   **Uterine contraction intensity** is the peak strength of the contraction. Intensity is determined by palpation or by internal electronic monitoring.

   **Palpation of uterine contraction intensity or tone** uses the finger tips to evaluate the contraction strength. Mild contractions permit the uterine fundus to be easily indented with the finger tips during the peak (strongest part) of the contraction. Moderate uterine contractions permit the fundus to be indented during the peak by the fingertips with difficulty. Strong uterine contractions do not permit the fundus to be indented at the peak by the fingertips.

   **Resting tone** is relaxation of the uterus between uterine contractions and is determined by palpation even when internal electronic monitoring technology is being used in order to verify the accuracy of the monitoring device (and especially when external monitoring is used).

   **Internal electronic monitoring** determines intensity of uterine contractions by using a pressure-sensitive intrauterine catheter to record the intensity and resting tone of uterine contractions in mm of Hg. The usual intensity of uterine contractions at the peak is 50-75 mm Hg during active labor.

   **Uterine contraction frequency, duration, and resting time** are recorded on the electronic monitoring strip in the external (tocodynamometer) mode and the internal (intrauterine catheter) mode. **Figure 15** is a tracing of uterine contractions indicating frequency, duration, intensity, and resting time.

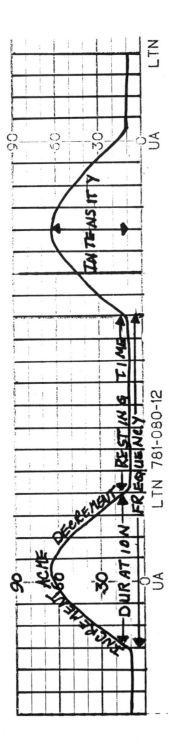

**Figure 15.** Uterine Contraction Frequency, Duration, Intensity, Resting Time, and Testing Tone. The portions of the uterine contraction are labeled as the increment, acme, and decrement. The increment is the gradual increase in tone or strength of the contraction as it builds to the peak (acme) strength. The decrement is the gradual relaxation of the uterine contraction, which is followed by relaxation (resting tone) of the uterus for the period of time between contractions (resting time).

b. The **cervix** is assessed for dilatation and effacement using intravaginal palpation of the cervical os with the index and middle finger. Dilatation (opening of the cervical os) is recorded in centimeters and effacement (cervical thinning and shortening) is recorded in percent. The range of cervical dilatation is 0-10 cm and the range of effacement is 0%-100% (2 cm thick to <1 mm thick). The expected rate of cervical dilatation in active labor for the primigravida should occur at the rate of 1.2 cm per hour and for the multipara at 1.5 cm per hour.

c. The **station** of the fetal presenting part is assessed using intravaginal palpation with the index and middle finger. The station is recorded as the number of centimeters the fetal presenting part is above or below the level of the maternal ischial spines. Palpation of the presenting part at the level of the ischial spines is zero station and indicates the occurrence of engagement. The expected rate of descent of the fetal presenting part during active labor is 1 cm per hour for the primigravida and 2 cm per hour for the multipara.

d. The **membranes** are assessed for intactness. The status of the membranes can be determined by palpation of the membranes during vaginal exam and by testing of vaginal fluid with Nitrazine paper (tests pH of the fluid and turns blue if amniotic fluid is present).

When rupture of the membranes occurs, the fetal heart rate is immediately assessed to detect evidence of prolapsed cord. The color and character of the amniotic fluid are assessed. The usual color is clear (meconium-stained fluid is greenish or greenish-yellow and indicates fetal hypoxia of a fetus with a cephalic presentation). The fluid is thin (watery) and has no offensive odor. Foul odor and/or thick fluid indicates potential for chorioamnionitis.

3. **Fetal well-being assessment** involves assessment of the fetal heart rate, presenting part presentation and position, and fetal movement. A summary of each component follows:

a. The **fetal heart rate** range is 120-160 bpm. Data can be obtained by auscultation or from the electronic fetal monitoring (EFM) strip.

Leopold's maneuvers (specific abdominal palpation technique to identify fetal position) are performed before auscultation or placement of the external ultrasound transducer for external EFM of the fetal heart rate. When EFM is used, additional data such as fetal heart rate patterns and variability can be evaluated to determine adequacy of respiratory reserve or potential fetal distress.

Fetal tachycardia (FHR >160 bpm for at least 10 minutes) may be caused by maternal fever (infection), fetal hypoxia, drugs (atropine, ritodrine), fetal anemia or cardiac arrhythmias, or maternal disorders. The occurrence of tachycardia is evaluated in terms of FHR patterns, baseline variability, and cause.

Bradycardia (FHR <120 bpm for at least 10 minutes) may be caused by worsening fetal hypoxia or development of fetal asphyxia, anesthesia drugs, maternal hypotension, umbilical cord compression, or fetal cardiac arrhythmia. The cause should be identified and the bradycardia evaluated in terms of baseline variability and the FHR pattern that occurs with the bradycardia.

b. The **fetal presenting part** is assessed during vaginal exam. Data are obtained regarding presentation and position to evaluate the potential for the passenger to successfully pass through the passage.

c. **Fetal movement** is assessed and evaluated to identify early signs of hypoxia (may be preceded by increased fetal movement) or signs of fetal distress (greatly decreased or absent fetal movement) or fetal demise (absent fetal movement).

4. **Maternal psychological well-being assessment** involves assessment of ability to cope with the discomfort of labor. Data to be evaluated include interaction with nurses and support persons, nonverbal behavior, as well as, the mother's verbaliza- tion of expectations and level of comfort and fatigue.

# ON-GOING MATERNAL AND FETAL WELL-BEING ASSESSMENT

**Maternal and fetal well-being and labor progress assessments** occur throughout the birthing process. Standards of care provide guidelines for frequency of assessment. During the latent phase recommendations are for maternal and fetal well-being assessment procedures to be performed every hour. During the active phase of labor, recommendations are for assessments to be performed every 30 minutes. Recommendations for the second stage are for assessments to be completed every 15 minutes. If the mother is classified as high-risk, recommendations are for latent phase assessment every 30 minutes, active phase every 15 minutes, and second stage every 5 minutes. Individual institutional policies usually require assessment similar to the recommendations or more frequently. Many institutions require continuous monitoring of the high-risk mother. Components of well-being assessment include maternal assessment and fetal assessment.

## Maternal Assessment

Maternal assessment components include the following:

1. **Vital signs** assessments include blood pressure, pulse and respirations usually occurring every hour during the latent phase, every 30 minutes during the active and transition phases, and every 15 minutes during the second stage for low-risk laboring mothers.

   If membranes are intact and the mother is afebrile, temperature is usually assessed every 4 hours. If the temperature is elevated (>37.5 degrees C) or if the membranes rupture, assessment is usually every hour throughout the birthing process.

2. **Uterine contractions** are assessed for frequency, duration, intensity, and resting time/tone at least every hour during the latent phase, at least every 30 minutes during the active phase, and at least every 15 minutes during the second stage for low-risk laboring mothers. It is common practice to assess uterine contractions each time the FHR is assessed because the FHR pattern is evaluated based on the response to uterine contractions.

3. **Labor progress** is assessed in terms of cervical dilatation and effacement, and fetal presenting part descent. The timing of the assessments is based on objective signs of labor progress. Objective signs include maternal nonverbal behavior, uterine contraction status, bloody show, rupture of membranes, maternal perceptions of perineal/rectal pressure, and characteristics of the FHR pattern. Once the membranes rupture, vaginal exams are minimized. Labor progress data are often recorded on the labor graph (Friedman graph) in order to evaluate progress and identify arrests in the birthing process.

   Cervical dilatation and fetal presenting part descent are plotted on the labor graph and compared to the dilatation and descent curves for the average progress for primigravid mothers or multiparous mothers.

4. **Membrane status** is assessed with each vaginal exam (see assessment notations above). The risk for chorioamnionitis increases with rupture of the membranes because of ascending bacteria from the vagina. Thus, it is desirable for birth to occur soon after the membranes rupture (within 12-24 hours). FHR assessment is monitored for verification of fetal well-being for several minutes following membranes rupture. If prolapsed cord is suspected, a vaginal exam is performed to palpate for the cord.

5. **Elimination** or bladder status is evaluated frequently (at least every two hours). The laboring mother may not distinguish full bladder from uterine contraction discomfort. A full bladder can

impede fetal presenting part descent. If the mother is unable to void, catheterization for distention is required.

## Fetal Assessment

**Fetal well-being assessment** recommendations include assessment of FHR range and pattern at least every hour during the latent phase, at least every 30 minutes during the active phase, and at least every 15 minutes during the second stage for the low-risk mother and fetus. As with maternal well-being assessment, individual institutions may modify the recommendations for more frequent assessment. Many institutions use continuous EFM of the low-risk mother/fetus as well as the high-risk mother/fetus throughout the birthing process. Often hospital policies recommend auscultation or EFM strip evaluation of the FHR range and pattern with each uterine contraction during the second stage of labor. The timing of fetal presentation and position assessment is based on objective signs of labor progress. Components of the on-going fetal well-being assessment for the low-risk fetus includes the following:

1. **FHR range of 120-160 bpm.** See notations above for fetal tachycardia or fetal bradycardia.

2. **FHR pattern** in response to uterine contractions are evaluated to identify reassuring or nonreassuring patterns.

   Characteristics of reassuring patterns include a baseline rate of 120-160 bpm, presence of short-term variability, average long-term variability, accelerations with fetal movement or uterine contractions, early decelerations, and mild or moderate variable decelerations (review notations in prenatal EFM assessment).

   Characteristics of nonreassuring patterns include loss of variability, late decelerations, severe variable decelerations, and tachycardiac or bradycardic baseline, especially with loss of variability (review notations in Selected Intrapartal Complications).

3. **Fetal presentation and position** are assessed with vaginal exams to verify achievement of the mechanisms of labor and to identify arrests in descent.

# IMMEDIATE NEONATAL ASSESSMENT

Assessment of the neonate immediately following birth begins with assessment for establishing respirations. Because the first minutes following birth are critical, the Apgar scoring system was developed to assess and document neonatal status at 1 and 5 minutes of age. Following completion of the Apgar assessment, a brief physical exam to identify gross abnormalities and to document vital sign stability is performed. Beginning family relationship is also assessed. A

summary of each component of the immediate neonatal assessment
follows:

1. **Apgar scoring** assesses five signs or parameters and assigns
   a value of 0, 1, or 2 to each parameter. The maximum score is
   10, and the score obtained documents the physiological status of
   the neonate at the time of completion of the scoring procedure.
   The usual score is 8-9 at 1 minute and 9 at 5 minutes and indicates the neonate is in good condition and requires warmth,
   suctioning and "blow-by" oxygen. A total score of 4-7 indicates
   respiratory depression and the need for airway clearance, stimulation and supplemental oxygen. A score below 4 is indicative of
   the need for resuscitation and/or CPR.

   The 5 parameters are heart rate, respiration, muscle tone, reflex,
   irritability, and color.

   Values assigned to heart rate are 0 for no heart beat, 1 for apical
   heart rate below 100 bpm, and 2 for apical heart rate above 100
   bpm.

   Values assigned to respirations are 0 for absence of respiratory
   effort, 1 for irregular or slow effort, and 2 for crying.

   Values assigned to muscle tone are 0 if the tone is flaccid, 1 for
   some flexion of the extremities, and 2 for good flexion or motion
   of the extremities.

   Values for reflex irritability are 0 for no response to stimulus
   (catheter inserted in the nostril or slapping the sole of the foot),
   1 for a facial grimace in response to stimulus, or 2 for crying in
   response to stimulus.

   Values for color are 0 for blue or pale color, 1 for a pink body and
   blue extremities (especially feet and hands), and 2 for pink body
   and extremities.

2. Brief physical assessment includes assessment of the following:
   a. Vital signs:
      Heart rate (120-160 bpm)

      - Respiration (30-60 rpm)

      - Temperature (axillary 97.6-98.7° F.; first temperature is
        often taken rectally to determine anal patency)

   b. Skin (color, staining, peeling, vernix caseosa)
   c. Head:
      - Circumference

      - Fontanelles (size; flat, full, bulging)

      - Molding

      - Caput succedaneum

- Cephalhematoma
- Mouth and palates
- Eyes (symmetry, hemorrhage, opacity)
- Nasal patency
- Ears (normal, low set)

**d.** Chest:
- Circumference
- Palpation of PMI (Point of Maximum Impulse)
- Auscultation of lung sounds
- Auscultation of heart sounds
- Size of breast bud

**e.** Abdomen:
- Number of vessels in cord (2 arteries, 1 vein)
- Umbilical hernia

**f.** Neurologic System:
- Reflexes (Moro, suck, root, Babinski, plantar and hand grasp)

**g.** Extremities:
- Ortolani's maneuver ("hip click")
- Sole creases

**h.** Genitalia

**i.** Length

**j.** Weight

3. **Vital signs** and color are assessed frequently, every 30-60 minutes, during the first 4 hours of life.

4. **Beginning relationship development** is evaluated by observing parental reaction to sex, size, and appearance of the neonate. Verbal and nonverbal behavior indicating acceptance (eye-to-eye contact, touching, naming) of the neonate provide a basis for nursing intervention to promote development of family relationships.

# CHAPTER 9

# NURSING INTERVENTION

*Nursing intervention for intrapartal mothers involves promotion of comfort, maintaining physiological functioning, and ensuring safety. Interventions for alterations in the birthing process for the mother and fetus are included in the intrapartal unit chapter 3, "Selected Intrapartal Complications."*

## PROMOTION OF COMFORT

**Promotion of comfort** involves nursing interventions focused on maternal physical and psychological comfort. Support persons are able to participate effectively in promoting comfort for the intrapartal mother.

### Physical Comfort

Physical comfort measures include hygiene, fluid intake, elimination, position, relaxation, and pain relief. Each measure is summarized below:

1. **Hygiene measures** focus on eliminating minor discomforts related to diaphoresis and vaginal discharge (amniotic fluid, bloody show) common during labor. By eliminating such minor discomforts, the mother is able to focus her energy on coping with the discomfort of uterine contractions instead of dividing her focus between labor discomfort and the other discomforts.

   Hygiene measures include such general hygiene activities as showers or Jacuzzi baths, clean/dry linens and gown, oral hygiene, removal of discharge from the vulva, changing Chux often, application of cool washcloths to the face, arranging hair comfortably, and offering handwashing often (especially following elimination).

2. **Fluid intake** prevents dehydration and relieves the discomfort of dry oral mucous membranes that occur because of use of various breathing patterns during labor. Fluid intake can be in the form of intravenous therapy, clear liquids by mouth, or a combination of both. If the mother is NPO, she and her support persons must be given an explanation for the order. Often ice chips or moist 4X4s are permitted with NPO status.

3. **Elimination**, especially bladder elimination, facilitates descent of the fetal presenting part by avoiding the barrier of a full bladder. In addition, a full bladder intensifies maternal discomfort. Remind the mother to void about every 2 hours. If bladder distention occurs and the mother is unable to void, catheterization will need

to be performed according to hospital policy and physician orders. Remember to insert the catheter between uterine contractions.

4. **Position changes/choices** permit the laboring mother to identify her own position of comfort. She needs to be able to change position often to prevent added discomfort due to maintaining the same position. In addition, walking, sitting in the rocking chair, squatting beside the bed, and/or assuming the "all fours" position permit the mother to find ever-changing positions of comfort as the fetus negotiates the birth canal and places pressure on different maternal structures. Remember to help the mother to avoid supine hypotension (elevate head of bed, place wedge under the right buttock) and avoid stress on extremities (slightly flex the joints).

5. **Relaxation techniques** include distraction (early in labor), imaging, patterned breathing techniques, music, focusing on a focal point, and/or shower or Jacuzzi bath. For the mother who has not participated in childbirth education classes, slow, deep breathing throughout labor, attendance of a supportive nurse and/or support person, and focusing on a favorite vacation spot can promote relaxation.

6. **Pain relief measures** include back rubs, counter pressure to the sacrum (especially for "back labor"), effleurage, analgesia, and anesthesia.

   a. **Back rubs** by the support person or nurse provide an opportunity to evaluate muscle tension as well as promote comfort and caring through touch.

   b. **Counter pressure** to the sacral area with the fist or an object such as a tennis ball promotes relief of back pain due to a fetus in the posterior position.

   c. **Effleurage** is light, rhythmic stroking of the abdomen with the finger tips by the mother or support person and promotes abdominal muscle relaxation.

   d. **Analgesia** involves the use of drugs to reduce the perception or sensation of pain. The classification of pain reducing drugs administered during labor include narcotics (Demerol), mixed narcotic agonist-antagonists (Stadol, Nubain), and analgesic potentiating drugs (Phenergan, Largon, Vistaril, Sparine). Analgesic drugs are most often administered IV because of the rapid onset of effect.

   The disadvantage of analgesic drugs is the respiratory depression effect on the neonate. CNS depression due to narcotic administration can be reversed by administration of a narcotic antagonist (Narcan, Trexan).

e. Anesthesia for labor includes administration of local anesthetic drugs (Xylocaine, Marcaine, Nesacaine, Pontocaine, Carbocaine). The effect of the anesthesia depends on the type of block used and the timing of administration. Each type has advantages and disadvantages which can help the mother choose which type she prefers. The types used for vaginal birth include local infiltration of the perineal area, pudendal block, saddle block, and lumbar epidural. Types of anesthesia used for cesarean birth include lumbar epidural and spinal block.

An additional type of anesthesia that is sometimes used for cesarean birth is general anesthesia. The disadvantages of general anesthesia are that the mother is not awake, risk of respiratory depression of mother and neonate, potential for vomiting and aspiration, and risk for uterine relaxation (which can result in postpartal atony and hemorrhage).

## Psychological Comfort

Psychological comfort measures include reduction of anxiety, planning for achievement of maternal goals, providing opportunities for choice, and respecting maternal focus during contractions. Suggested measures to promote psychological comfort are summarized below:

1. **Reduction of anxiety** measures include educational preparation for the birthing process, explanation of all procedures, listening to the mother's concerns and fears, remaining with the mother throughout labor, praising the mother's coping efforts, and verbally expressing confidence in the mother's ability to successfully complete the birthing process. In addition, explaining what labor changes/events that can be expected next (such as the characteristics of the next phase or stage) can help the mother and her support persons to be prepared and avoid fear of inability to cope with the sensations and discomforts of each phase and stage of labor.

2. **Achievement of maternal goals** measures include fulfilling the role of client advocate, and verifying with the mother her desire to continue the process as she planned. For example, the mother may have a goal of not using analgesia as a coping technique for discomfort. As labor progresses, the nurse needs to verify that the mother desires to strive to achieve the goal. If the mother decides to continue the process without use of analgesia, the nurse may need to serve as a patient advocate with support persons and/or physician who want the mother to accept the analgesia.

3. **Maternal choice** permits the mother to maintain some level of control over a process that seems to be overwhelming and never ending. Since the mother has no choice over the physiological

events that occur, permitting her to make as many choices as possible will reinforce her perception of herself as a person rather than an object. For example, giving her the choice of ambulating to the bathroom or using the bedpan to empty her bladder or choosing a position of comfort reinforce control at some level. Another example is protecting maternal modesty.

4. **Maternal focus** during uterine contractions can be maintained by performing all nursing interventions and assessment procedures between uterine contractions rather than during contractions. Disruption of maternal focus/concentration on her chosen relaxation technique is frustrating and intensifies the physical discomfort felt by the mother. It also intensifies her feeling of lack of control over any part of the process.

# MAINTAINING PHYSIOLOGIC FUNCTIONING

Intervention measures to support **maintenance of physiologic functioning** involve evaluating maternal and fetal response to the birthing process, performing nursing actions based on evaluation of maternal and fetal response, and promoting rest between uterine contractions. Examples of intervention measures to support physiologic functioning include change of maternal position based on FHR response or fetal presenting part position, administration of oxygen by mask based on FHR response, and increasing the mainline IV flow rate based on maternal and/or fetal response.

## Ensuring Safety

**Ensuring maternal and fetal safety** measures focus on preventing trauma or adverse outcomes. Examples of nursing interventions to promote safety include, recognizing a full bladder and emptying it before overdistention and potential for injury occur, raising the side-rails to prevent falls, assisting the mother to the bathroom, assessing for cord prolapse following rupture of the membranes, and using aseptic technique for vaginal exams, venipuncture, and catheterizations.

# CHAPTER 10

# SELECTED INTRAPARTAL COMPLICATIONS

*Intrapartal complications can be anticipated in the mother and the pregnancy classified as being high risk due to preexisting medical conditions or gestational conditions. However, complications can also occur suddenly. Because of the sudden occurrence of problems and because two lives are involved, careful nursing assessment, decision-making, and intervention are essential. "Selected Intrapartal Complications" involves some of the more commonly experienced problems that can occur during the birthing process. The problems have been categorized as problems with the passage, passenger, power, placenta, physiology, or maternal psychology. Finally, two treatment methods for intrapartal complications are summarized.*

## PROBLEMS WITH THE PASSAGE

**Problems with the passage** involve the pelvis and soft tissues. Definitions, outcomes, symptoms, consequences, assessment, and interventions for each of the problems are summarized below.

### Problems with the Pelvis

**Problems with the pelvis** include diminished inlet, midpelvis, and/or outlet pelvic diameters. Diminished maternal pelvic diameters interfere with passage of an at least average-sized fetus.

1. **Pelvic inlet contracture** is defined as an inlet in which the shortest anteroposterior diameter measures less than 10 cm or the longest transverse diameter measures less than 12 cm (Olds, London, Ladewig, 1996).

   The outcome for inlet contracture is inability of the fetal presenting part to engage (because of cephalopelvic disproportion) and an increased risk for umbilical cord prolapse.

   a. Symptoms of inlet contracture include:

   **Subjective:**

   – Verbalization of difficult breathing (due to high fundus)

   – Verbalization of sore ribs (due to high fundus)

**Objective:**

- Failure of presenting part to engage

- Abnormal presentation (face, shoulder)

- Weak contractions may occur

b. Consequences for the fetus include extreme molding of the head and potential trauma, risk of fetal hypoxia/asphyxia with prolapse of the umbilical cord when membranes rupture (due to unengagement of the presenting part), and trauma due to malposition.

Maternal consequences of inlet contracture include prolonged labor, risk of uterine rupture, and trauma to soft tissues.

c. Assessment for inlet contracture includes assessment of fetal presentation, fetal position, fetal lie, maternal pelvis adequacy, size of the fetus, and fetal station.

d. Intervention measures for inlet contracture include education of the mother regarding the progress of labor, the underlying cause of the problem, the potential risks, medical interventions, and the expected outcomes. Additional interventions include frequent change of maternal position, suggesting positions that increase the pelvic diameters (such as squatting), promoting maternal and fetal well-being, and providing maternal emotional support.

2. **Midpelvic contracture** is defined as a value of 13.5 cm or less for the sum of the interischial spine diameter and the posterior sagittal diameter (Bobak and Jensen, 1993).

The outcome of midpelvic contracture is arrest of fetal descent.

a. Symptoms of midpelvic contracture include the following:

**Objective:**

- Failure of fetal presenting part descent

- Persistent fetal presenting part transverse position

b. Fetal consequences of midpelvic contracture are similar to those for inlet contracture. Maternal consequences may be cesarean birth.

c. Assessment is the same as for inlet contracture assessment.

d. Intervention is the same as for inlet contracture intervention.

3. **Outlet pelvic contracture** is defined as an interischial diameter measurement of 8 cm or less (Bobak and Jensen, 1993).

The outcome for outlet pelvic contracture is arrest of fetal descent. Outlet pelvic contractures are often associated with midpelvic contractures and the male-type pelvis.

a. Symptoms of outlet pelvic contracture include the following:

**Objective:**

- Narrow maternal pubic arch

- Arrest in descent of the fetal presenting part

b. Fetal consequences of outlet pelvic contracture are similar to those for inlet contracture. Maternal consequences include increased risk of maternal soft tissue lacerations if vaginal birth does occur.

c. Assessment is the same as for inlet contracture assessment.

d. Intervention is the same as for inlet contracture intervention.

## Problems with the Soft Tissues

**Problems with the soft tissues** involve soft tissue barriers, rupture of the uterus, and inversion of the uterus. Each soft tissue problem is summarized as follows:

1. **Soft tissue barriers** most commonly include a full bladder and full rectum. Occasionally fibroid tumors, ovarian tumors, or a pathological retraction ring (Bandl's ring) may occur and block fetal presenting part descent.

   The pathologic retraction ring usually occurs during the second stage of labor (after the fetal head has passed through the cervix) as the wall of the upper uterine segment thickens and the lower uterine segment wall remains thin. Normally, the junction between the thinning lower uterine segment and the thickening upper uterine segment remains flexible to permit passage of the fetus from the uterus. When pathology occurs, the junction constricts and prevents descent of the fetus.

   The outcome for soft tissue barriers is determined by options for removal of the barrier. Full bladder and full rectum are easily removed once they are diagnosed. Removal of fibroid or ovarian tumors are usually not an option during labor and may necessitate cesarean birth. The pathologic retraction ring must be recognized and intervention achieved before uterine rupture occurs.

   a. Symptoms of common soft tissue barriers are the following:

   **Full bladder**:

   - Bulge above the symphysis pubis

   **Full rectum:**

   - Bulge in the posterior vaginal area

**Pathologic retraction ring:**

- — Palpable uterine indentation
- — Arrest in fetal descent
- — Strong uterine contractions with no progress of labor

b. Consequences of full bladder and full rectum for the fetus include arrest in descent. Maternal consequences include increased maternal discomfort and potential trauma to maternal soft tissues.

c. Assessment activities for full bladder include careful notation of intake and urinary output in terms of amount and frequency, and palpation of the bladder in the lower abdominal area above the symphysis.

Assessment activities for full rectum include history regarding last bowel movement and usual bowel habits, and palpation of the fullness of the rectum through the vaginal wall on vaginal exam.

Assessment for pathologic retraction ring includes assessment for progression of labor/fetal descent and palpation of the uterus through the abdominal wall.

d. Intervention for full bladder includes assisting the mother to the bathroom or catheterization for inability to void.

Intervention for full rectum includes evacuation of the rectum.

Intervention for pathologic retraction ring includes notification of the physician, preparation for uterine relaxation and immediate cesarean birth, parental education regarding causes and consequences of the pathologic retraction ring, emotional support of the parents, and education of parents for cesarean birth.

2. **Uterine rupture** is a tearing of the myometrium (incomplete) or all 3 (complete) layers of the uterus. It is caused most often by separation of a previous scar (previous cesarean birth or other operative procedure) but can also be caused by trauma. Traumatic causes include:

- Mismanaged oxytocin infusion (tetanic contractions)
- Cephalopelvic disproportion (obstructed labor)
- Pathologic retraction ring (obstructed labor)
- Malpresentation of the fetus
- Traumatic maneuvers (external version, forceps, traction)

**a**. Symptoms

**Subjective:**

- Maternal complaints of sudden severe pain (complete rupture)

- Possible maternal description of the pain as a tearing sensation (complete rupture)

- Maternal complaints of local tenderness (above site of incomplete rupture)

- Maternal complaints of aching pain (over the area in incomplete rupture)

**Objective:**

- Cessation of uterine contractions

- Palpation of separate fetal and uterine masses (complete rupture)

- Signs of shock due to peritoneal hemorrhage (complete rupture)

- Cessation of FHR (complete rupture)

- Gradual development of maternal distress (incomplete rupture)

- Gradual development of fetal distress (incomplete rupture with intact placenta)

**b.** Consequences of uterine rupture for the fetus include fetal distress due to interruption of blood supply to the uterus (even in incomplete rupture) and rapid fetal demise with complete rupture.

Maternal consequences include an increased risk for mortality, especially with complete rupture, and sterilization by tubal ligation or hysterectomy, especially with a severe rupture. In either case, future childbearing is not advised.

**c.** Assessment activities include monitoring for signs of causes of impending uterine rupture, careful review of maternal history for risk factors of uterine rupture, careful assessment of maternal and fetal response to intravenous oxytocin, and assessment of maternal subjective data.

**d.** Intervention measures include notification of the physician, maintenance of maternal physiological stability (oxygen, fluids, medications), emotional support of the parents, explanation of the cause and consequences, timely information regarding fetal well-being and outcome, and grief counseling (fetal loss, fertility loss).

3. **Uterine inversion** occurs rarely and involves the turning of the uterus "inside out." It is caused by application of pressure to the fundus or traction on an attached placenta when the uterus is relaxed. Fundal pressure to assist with delivery of the placenta or excessive fundal pressure in a relaxed uterus to control postdelivery blood loss can precipitate inversion. Traction on the umbilical cord of an attached placenta due to short umbilical cord as the fetus is born or intentional traction on the cord to hasten delivery of the placenta can result on inversion of the relaxed uterus.

Outcome of uterine inversion depends on the rapidity with which the uterus is replaced. Maternal risk for blood loss and death increase with every minute of time between inversion and replacement.

a. Symptoms

   – Sudden increase in vaginal bleeding

   – No fundus palpable abdominally

   – Continued vaginal blood loss

   – Signs of shock

b. Consequences of uterine inversion for the fetus is usually not applicable since it occurs after birth of the fetus.

   Maternal consequences include hemorrhage and increased risk for maternal death, if the uterus cannot be replaced quickly so that it can contract and control blood loss.

c. Assessment activities include careful assessment of uterine tone before applying fundal pressure, assessment for signs of uterine inversion, and assessment of maternal physiologic response to the third and fourth stages of labor.

d. Intervention measures include maintenance of maternal physiological stability, preparation of mother for immediate general anesthesia to effect relaxation for uterine replacement, explanation of events to mother and support person, and provision of emotional support.

# PROBLEMS WITH THE PASSENGER

**Problems with the passenger** involve presentation, position, size, and distress. Problems are summarized as follows:

## Problems with Fetal Presentation

**Problems with fetal presentation** include breech presentation, face or brow presentation, and transverse lie (shoulder presentation). Fetal malpresentations are summarized as follows:

1. **Breech presentation** involves the breech as the presenting part rather than the head. The types of breech presentation are the complete breech (thighs flexed on abdomen, knees flexed with calves flexed on thighs, feet and buttocks as presenting parts), frank breech (knees extended, thighs flexed on abdomen, calves extended on chest, buttocks as presenting part), single or double footling breech (one or both feet as the presenting part), and kneeling breech (knee as the presenting part).

   Breech presentation occurs with preterm labor, small fetus (<2500 g), placenta previa or fibroid tumor blocking entrance to the pelvis, lax maternal abdominal muscles (multiparity), hydramnios, hydrocephalus, oligohydramnios, uterine anomalies, or multiple gestation.

   The outcome for breech presentation often involves cesarean birth to reduce potential perinatal mortality and morbidity.

   a. Symptoms include:

   – Palpation of the fetal head in the fundus

   – Auscultation of the FHR above the umbilicus

   – Palpation of the breech in the lower uterine segment

   – Meconium-stained amniotic fluid during labor (due to compression of the fetal intestinal tract)

   b. Consequences of breech presentation for the fetus include preterm birth, increased risk of perinatal morbidity and mortality due to prolapsed cord or cord compression, CPD of the unmolded aftercoming head, birth trauma, and neurologic abnormalities that may not become apparent until later in life.

   Maternal consequences include the potential for a longer labor when vaginal birth is permitted, since the breech is not as effective in dilating the cervix as the head, and a cesarean birth.

   c. Assessment for breech presentation includes performance of Leopold's maneuvers, location of site of FHR auscultation, identification of presenting part(s) on vaginal exam, and careful assessment of fetal well-being if vaginal birth is attempted.

   d. Intervention includes education of the parents regarding vaginal birth for breech, external version procedure, or cesarean birth for breech; preparation for external version, vaginal breech delivery, or cesarean section; parental support; and provision of ongoing fetal well-being information to the parents.

2. **Brow or Face presentation** is extension rather than flexion of the fetal head with the brow or face as the presenting part. Brow/Face presentation occurs more often with preterm labor,

fetal head anomalies, placenta previa, contracted pelvis, or multi-parity.

Outcome for brow/face presentation depends on the size of the maternal pelvis and the size of the fetal head. Usually the diameters presented by the fetal head to the maternal pelvis in the brow/face presentation are too large for the mechanisms of labor to occur because of CPD. Cesarean birth is a frequent outcome.

   a. Symptoms include:

   – Abdominal palpation of the extended fetal head on the same side as the back

   – Auscultation of the FHR on the side of the fetal extremities (through the chest versus back)

   – Palpation of the anterior fontanelle and brow or facial structures on vaginal exam

   – Delay in engagement or failure of engagement to occur

   b. Consequences of brow/face presentation for the fetus include trauma to the face and CPD. Maternal consequences include prolonged labor or cesarean section for CPD.

   c. Assessment for brow/face presentation includes careful performance of Leopold's maneuvers, identification of the presenting part on vaginal exam, and assessment of maternal and fetal well-being.

   d. Intervention measures for brow/face presentation include education of parents regarding the impact of the presentation on labor and birth, preparation for cesarean birth (if CPD occurs), maternal emotional support and comfort for a longer labor, and education of parents for appearance of the neonatal face (petechiae, ecchymosis, edema).

3. **Transverse lie** (shoulder presentation) occurs in women with lax abdominal muscles (multiparity), contracted pelvic inlet, fibroid tumors in the lower uterine segment, placenta previa, hydramnios, preterm labor, hydrocephaly or other anomalies that prevent engagement, and multiple gestation.

   Outcome for transverse lie at term is usually cesarean birth.

   a. Symptoms of transverse lie include:

   – Fundal height less than dates would indicate

   – Lateral width of the uterus is greater than fundal height

   – Palpation of shoulder or arm as the presenting part on vaginal exam

**b.** Consequences of transverse lie for the fetus include risk for prolapsed cord (with rupture of membranes because the presenting part does not block the inlet), and risk for morbidity and mortality due to fetal asphyxia and trauma.

Maternal consequences of transverse lie include anxiety regarding fetal well-being, disappointment in not being able to achieve a vaginal birth, cesarean birth, and risk for uterine rupture.

**c.** Assessment activities include careful performance of Leopold's maneuvers, abdominal inspection, fundal height assessment, location of FHTs, and vaginal exam.

**d.** Intervention measures involve notification of the physician of the assessment findings, careful assessment for prolapsed cord with rupture of membranes, education of the parents regarding the presentation and cesarean birth, emotional support of the parents, maintenance of maternal and fetal well-being, and preparation for cesarean birth.

## Problems with Fetal Position

**Problems with fetal position** include persistent occiput posterior position and transverse arrest. Malposition may occur in women with other than gynecoid pelves or contracted pelves. Each malposition is summarized as follows:

**1. Persistent occiput posterior** is the most common fetal malposition. Instead of rotating anteriorly during the internal rotation mechanism, the occiput rotates posteriorly (or remains posterior if descent began in the posterior position).

Outcome may be a forcep or vacuum assisted birth or a cesarean birth if rotation does not occur and descent is arrested.

**a.** Symptoms of persistent posterior position include the following:

**Subjective:**

– Complaints of severe back pain

**Objective:**

– Observation of a depression in the abdominal curve above the symphysis pubis

– Auscultation of FHR in the far lateral quadrant

– Dysfunctional labor pattern

– Prolonged active phase

– Arrest in descent

- Prolonged second stage
- Occiput posterior position on vaginal exam

b. Consequences of persistent occiput posterior position for the fetus include potential for cesarean birth if vaginal delivery cannot be effected.

The consequences for the mother include prolonged labor, maternal exhaustion, risk for postpartal hemorrhage (due to uterine exhaustion), risk for third or fourth degree laceration, and potential for cesarean birth.

c. Assessment activities for persistent occiput posterior position include careful assessment for subjective and objective symptoms, full bladder, and labor progression.

d. Intervention measures for persistent occiput posterior position include explanation for the back pain and prolonged labor, comfort measures (counter pressure to the sacrum, frequent change of position, "all fours" position, pelvic rock, squatting for second stage) to stimulate fetal head rotation, emotional support, and preparation for operative birth (forceps or vacuum rotation, or cesarean).

## Problems with Fetal Size

**Problems with fetal size** usually involve fetuses that weigh at least 4000 g (8 lbs 13 ozs, classified as macrosomic) or hydrocephaly. Each problem is summarized as follows:

1. **Macrosomia** is often caused by maternal diabetes mellitus. Other causes include maternal obesity, excessive maternal weight gain during the pregnancy, multiparity, and postterm pregnancy.

Outcome for macrosomia is often cesarean birth due to CPD and/or shoulder dystocia.

a. Symptoms include the following:

- Fundal height greater than dates
- Abdominal palpation of a large baby
- Delayed engagement
- Arrest in descent
- Dysfunctional labor pattern (due to overdistended uterus)

b. Consequences of macrosomia for the fetus include potential trauma, asphyxia, fractured clavicle, and brachial plexus injury if macrosomia is not recognized.

Maternal consequences include prolonged labor, potential postpartal hemorrhage (due to uterine atony), or cesarean birth.

c. Assessment activities for macrosomia include careful review of maternal history for risk factors, Leopold's maneuvers, labor progression, maternal well-being, and fetal well-being.

d. Intervention measures for macrosomia include maintenance of maternal and fetal physiological well-being, emotional support, explanation of macrosomia and the potential for cesarean birth, and preparation for vaginal or cesarean birth.

2. **Hydrocephaly** is enlargement of the fetal cranium due to accumulation of excess cerebrospinal fluid in the ventricles and subarachnoid spaces of the brain.

Outcome of hydrocephaly depends on the occurrence of other fetal anomalies commonly associated with the hydrocephaly, the degree of impairment and threat to life caused by the anomalies, and the viability of the fetus. Cesarean birth presents the least amount of trauma to the fetus.

a. Symptoms of hydrocephaly include:

- Large fetal head palpated on Leopold's maneuvers

- Delayed or failure of engagement

- Wide fetal skull sutures on vaginal exam

b. Consequences of hydrocephaly for the fetus include an increased mortality rate due to brain damage and/or other accompanying fetal anomalies.

Maternal consequences include increased risk for cesarean birth and obstruction of labor with increased risk of uterine rupture if hydrocephaly is not recognized.

c. Assessment activities for hydrocephaly include Leopold's maneuvers, vaginal exam, and parental perception and understanding of hydrocephaly and its consequences.

d. Intervention measures for hydrocephaly include emotional parental support, parental education, parental preparation for vaginal or cesarean birth, and preparation for parental grieving support.

## Problems with Fetal Distress

**Fetal distress** is insufficient fetal oxygenation usually due to placental insufficiency or cord compression. Placental insufficiency can be caused by maternal medical disorder, placental anomaly, or fetal anomaly.

Outcome for fetal distress depends on the type (acute, chronic, or a combination), the severity, the ability to correct the problem, and the amount of time between diagnosis and birth (if the problem cannot be corrected).

1. Symptoms of potential fetal distress include meconium-stained amniotic fluid and FHR patterns that cannot be considered as reassuring. Fetal distress is diagnosed by documentation of acidosis based on blood pH.

    a. Symptoms of nonreassuring FHR patterns present a warning of deteriorating fetal well-being and include the following (see **Figure 16 and 17):**

    – Progressive FHR baseline increase or decrease

    – Progressive decrease in FHR variability

    – Tachycardia (FHR 160 bpm or more)

    – Severe variable decelerations

    – Late decelerations

    – Loss of variability

    – Prolonged deceleration

    – Severe bradycardia

    **Note:** Severe variable decelerations are those with a FHR below 60 bpm (or a decrease in FHR of 60 bpm from baseline) and lasting 60 seconds or longer (Olds et. al., 1996; Lowdermilk, Perry & Bobak, 1997). In addition, they are usually accompanied by decrease in variability, slow return to baseline FHR, and possibly an overshoot (rebound acceleration) on return to baseline.

    A prolonged deceleration lasts 120 seconds or longer.

    b. Diagnostic symptoms of fetal distress include the following:

    – Fetal scalp blood pH of 7.20-7.24 indicates preacidosis

    – Fetal scalp blood pH <7.20 indicates acidosis

Consequences of fetal distress for the fetus include potential mental retardation, potential for cerebral palsy, and a greater risk for fetal demise. Maternal consequences include anxiety regarding fetal well-being.

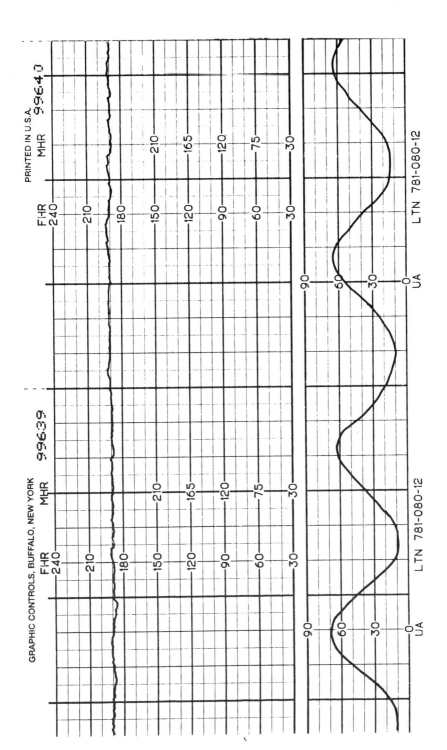

**Figure 16.** Nonreassuring FHR Pattern showing decreased variability and tachycardia.

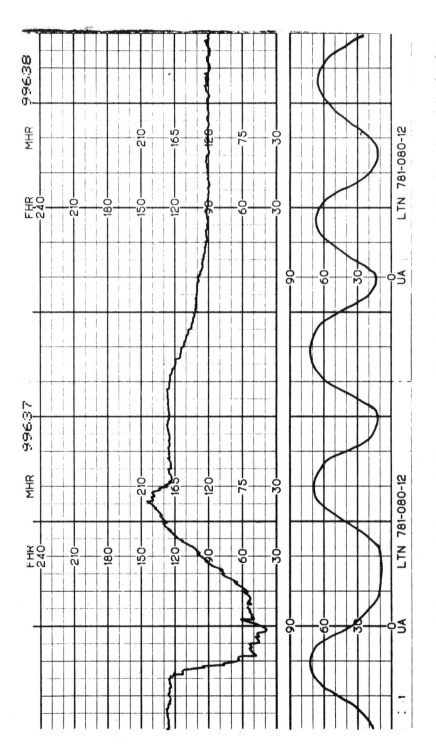

**Figure 17.** Potentially Ominous FHR Pattern showing a severe variable deceleration with overshoot and a prolonged deceleration. Note also the decrease in resting time between uterine contractions to less than 30 seconds.

2. Assessment activities for fetal distress include careful evaluation of maternal history for risk factors, monitoring of FHR patterns, maternal reports of sudden increase or decrease in fetal movements, assessment for prolapsed cord on vaginal exam, and assessment of amniotic fluid for color and consistency.

3. Intervention measures for fetal distress include change of maternal position (especially left lateral), administration of oxygen by mask to the mother, decrease or discontinue administration of oxytocin infusion, notify physician of FHR pattern, explain to parents the potential occurrence of fetal distress and rationale for corrective procedures, provide emotional support, and prepare for fetal scalp blood sampling and/or cesarean birth.

# PROBLEMS WITH THE POWER

**Problems with the power** involve the primary force (uterine contraction) that moves the passenger through the passage. The problems include dysfunctional labor patterns, prolonged labor, precipitous labor, preterm labor, and postterm labor.

## Problems with Dysfunctional Labor Patterns

**Problems with dysfunctional labor patterns** have been termed dystocia (a long and/or difficult labor). Dysfunctional labor patterns can be classified as hypertonic dysfunction or hypotonic dysfunction. Each classification is summarized below.

1. **Hypertonic dysfunctional labor pattern** has the following characteristics:

   - Increased resting tone (at least 15 mm Hg)

   - Increased contraction frequency

   - Decreased contraction intensity

   - Occurs in the latent phase (before 4 cm dilatation)

   - Very painful contractions (due to uterine muscle cell anoxia)

   - Ineffective contractions (no progression of cervical effacement or dilatation)

   The cause of hypertonic uterine dysfunction is thought to be uncoordinated uterine contractions (different muscle cells contracting independently rather than in a pattern) and/or origination of the force of the contraction in the uterine midsection rather than the fundus. Thus, the entire uterus is never relaxed (some part is contracting all the time).

   The profile of the mother experiencing hypertonic uterine dysfunction is often a very anxious primigravid mother at term or she may be postterm. The lack of resting time between uterine contractions interferes with her attempts to relax or use coping mechanisms with the discomfort.

Outcome can be a prolonged labor with adverse effects on mother and fetus, if the pattern does not convert to a more effective pattern or is not recognized and corrected. The usual method of correcting the pattern is to achieve rest, uterine relaxation, and maternal sleep through administration of analgesics. With uterine relaxation, an effective uterine contraction pattern often occurs spontaneously or can be initiated when the mother awakens.

a. Symptoms of hypertonic uterine dysfunction include the following:

**Subjective:**

- Very painful uterine contractions
- Verbalization of frustration
- Verbalization of ineffectiveness of relaxation techniques

**Objective:**

- Frequent uterine contractions
- Increased resting tone
- Decreased resting time
- Mild intensity
- Lack of progressive cervical change

b. Consequences of uncorrected hypertonic uterine dysfunction for the fetus include early fetal distress (due to lack of time for uteroplacental exchange), potential fetal demise (due to unrecognized asphyxia), excessive molding and/or trauma to the fetal head (due to prolonged pressure on the fetal head).

Maternal consequences of uncorrected hypertonic uterine dysfunction include potential for a prolonged latent phase, frustration because of being accused of overreacting to mild uterine contractions, discouragement due to lack of progress and perceived ineffectiveness of coping strategies, and increased anxiety regarding lack of progress.

c. Assessment activities for hypertonic uterine dysfunction include a careful history of the labor process and coping strategies before admission, assessment of resting tone and time, assessment of contraction pattern, cervical assessment, assessment of maternal/paternal emotional level, assessment of relaxation and coping strategies, and careful assessment of fetal well-being.

d. Intervention measures for hypertonic uterine dysfunction include explanation of the cause of the contraction pattern and planned correction, parental emotional support, promotion of rest and relaxation (environment, maternal position, medication), and a caring, accepting nursing attitude.

2. **Hypotonic dysfunctional labor pattern** has the following characteristics:

- Normal latent phase

- Normal initial active phase

- Progressive weakening of intensity of uterine contractions

- Progressive decrease in uterine contraction frequency (<2-3 contractions per 10 minute period)

- Possible cessation of uterine contractions

- Occurs after 4 cm dilatation

- Cervical change ceases

- Fetal descent ceases

The cause of hypotonic uterine dysfunction may be due to overstretching of the uterine muscle cells (macrosomia, multiple gestation, hydramnios), grand multiparity, early administration of analgesics (latent phase), fetal malposition, CPD, or contracted pelvis.

The profile of the mother experiencing hypotonic uterine dysfunction is often a multiparous mother in active labor.

Outcome in unrecognized and uncorrected hypotonic uterine dysfunction is prolonged labor and potential for intrauterine infection (if membranes have ruptured). The usual method of correction is to improve the quality of the uterine contractions (augmentation) once the adequacy of the pelvis is confirmed.

a. Symptoms of uncorrected hypotonic uterine dysfunction include:

**Subjective:**

– Painless uterine contractions

**Objective:**

– Uterine contractions (UCs) of decreasing intensity

– UC pattern of decreasing frequency or cessation

– Cessation of cervical change

– Cessation of fetal descent

   **b.** Consequences of uncorrected hypotonic uterine dysfunction for the fetus include distress due to potential intrauterine infection.

   Maternal consequences of uncorrected hypotonic uterine dysfunction include prolonged labor with risk of intrauterine infection (due to prolonged rupture of membranes), maternal exhaustion, emotional stress, and increased risk for postpartal hemorrhage (due to ineffective uterine contraction postpartum).

   **c. Assessment activities for hypotonic uterine dysfunction** include maternal vital signs, UC frequency and intensity, fetal well-being, symptoms of intrauterine infection (fever, chills, foul smelling amniotic fluid and/or change in color and character of the amniotic fluid), maternal hydration status, and maternal and support person coping strategies.

   **d.** Intervention measures for hypotonic uterine dysfunction include education regarding the cause and treatment of hypotonic uterine dysfunction, emotional support, preparation for oxytocin administration, and preparation for vaginal or cesarean birth.

## Problems with Prolonged Labor

**Problems with prolonged labor** can be defined in general as labor that lasts longer than 24 hours. Prolonged labor can occur because of prolonged latent phase, prolonged active phase, or prolonged descent. Each is summarized as follows:

1. **Prolonged latent phase** occurs when the latent phase lasts longer than 20 hours for a primigravida or 14 hours for a multipara. Prolonged latent phase can be caused by hypertonic uterine dysfunction, premature rupture of membranes with an unripe cervix, early administration of analgesia or anesthesia, or fetal malposition.

2. **Prolonged active phase** occurs when cervical dilatation in the primigravida is less than 1.2 cm per hour and less than 1.5 cm per hour in the multipara. Prolonged active phase may be caused by CPD, pelvic contracture(s), overdistended uterus, or maternal exhaustion.

3. **Prolonged descent** occurs when fetal descent in the active phase of labor is less than 1.0 cm per hour in a primigravida or 2.0 cm per hour in a multipara. Prolonged descent can be caused by full bladder, full rectum, maternal exhaustion, fetal malposition, CPD, pelvic contracture(s), or excessive use of analgesics or analgesia (causing a problem/compromise of secondary [bearing down] power).

Outcomes for prolonged labor include promotion of an effective labor pattern with vaginal birth or cesarean birth for CPD or failure to achieve an effective labor pattern.

   **a.** Symptoms of prolonged labor include some combination of those for hypertonic or hypotonic uterine dysfunction (see symptoms above) resulting in prolonged latent phase, active phase and/or descent.

   **b.** Consequences of prolonged labor for the fetus include fetal distress, increased risk of intrauterine infection, increased risk of prolapsed cord, and fetal head trauma.

   Maternal consequences of prolonged labor include maternal exhaustion, increased stress, increased risk of intrauterine infection and postpartal hemorrhage, and increased risk for operative delivery (forceps, vacuum extraction, cesarean).

   **c.** Assessment for prolonged labor includes assessment of maternal physiologic well-being, fetal well-being, UC pattern, cervical change, fetal presenting part descent, maternal coping, amniotic fluid color and character, and the effectiveness of treatment (rest, relaxation, augmentation).

   **d.** Intervention measures for prolonged labor include maintenance of maternal physiologic status (hydration, vital signs, comfort, hygiene) and fetal well-being (oxygenation), promotion of emotional support, facilitation of maternal relaxation, enhancement of maternal coping strategies, and promotion of maternal positions to improve descent (semi-Fowler's, squatting).

## Problems with Precipitous Labor

**Problems with precipitous labor** occur because of the short duration of labor (<3 hours from onset of UCs). Causes include excessively strong (tetanic-like) UCs (spontaneous or induced), lax maternal soft tissues (cervix, vagina, peritoneum) that present little resistance to dilatation and descent, multiparity, large pelvis, or a small fetus. Outcome, symptoms, consequences, assessment, and intervention for precipitous labor are summarized below:

   **1.** Outcome for precipitous labor is often emergency birth.

   **2.** Symptoms of precipitous labor include the following:

   **Subjective:**

- Painful UCs
- Sudden onset of UCs

**Objective:**

- Intense UCs

- Increased frequency of UCs

- 90 second or longer duration of UCs

- Decreased resting time (<30 seconds)

- Primigravida cervical dilatation >5 cm per hour

- Multipara cervical dilatation >10 cm per hour

- Rapid fetal presenting part descent

- Possible increased bloody show

3. Consequences of precipitous labor for the fetus include hypoxia (due to decreased uteroplacental exchange with decreased resting time), risk for intracranial hemorrhage (due to pressure exerted on the fetal head), and risk for brachial nerve plexus trauma.

   Maternal consequences of precipitous labor include increased risk for soft tissue lacerations (cervix, vagina, perineum, periurethral area), uterine rupture (due to tetanic UCs), amniotic fluid embolism, and postpartal hemorrhage.

4. Assessment activities for precipitous labor include frequent assessment of UC pattern, cervical change, presenting part descent, maternal physiological status, and fetal well-being (oxygenation and response to UCs).

5. Intervention measures for precipitous labor include constant nursing attendance, preparation for emergency delivery, discontinuing oxytocin for hyperstimulation/tetanic UCs (frequency >2 minutes, duration >90 seconds, resting time <30 seconds), left side-lying position, oxygen by mask, emotional support, and promotion of maternal relaxation.

## Problems with Preterm Labor

**Problems with preterm labor** involve the risk of birth of a premature neonate. The potential causes, outcome, and symptoms are presented in the prenatal unit (see Chapter 6: "Selected Prenatal Complications"). Assessment and intervention for progressive preterm labor and birth are summarized as follows:

1. Assessment activities for progressive preterm labor include frequent assessment of UC pattern and resting time, fetal well-being and response to labor (continuous electronic fetal monitoring), maternal physiological status, and maternal psychological/emotional status.

2. Intervention measures for progressive preterm labor include promotion of comfort, emotional support, positioning in the left side-lying position as often as possible, use of discomfort coping strategies other than analgesics (due to depressive effect on the fetus/neonate), and preparation for operative birth (episiotomy to shorten second stage and reduce pressure on fetal head, or cesarean for fetal distress or malpresentation).

## Problems with Postterm Labor

**Problems with postterm labor** occur because of the effect of a prolonged pregnancy, beyond 42 weeks gestation, on fetal well-being. The cause of true (versus faulty due-date estimation) postterm pregnancy is unknown but thought to be because the changes that initiate labor do not occur. The outcome, symptoms, consequences, assessment, and intervention for postterm labor are summarized as follows:

1. Outcome for postterm labor is induction of labor beyond 42 weeks gestation (or sooner if signs of decreased fetal reserve are indicated by nonstress or stress testing and/or biophysical profile).

2. Symptoms of postterm gestation include documentation of 42 weeks (or 294 days) since the LNMP by ultrasound dating of gestational age, 22 weeks of fetoscope positive auscultations, and size-date consistent fundal height measurements.

3. Consequences of postterm gestation for the fetus include fetal distress due to placental insufficiency ("old" placenta) and/or cord compression (due to oligohydramnios), birth trauma (due to macrosomia and/or shoulder dystocia), increased risk for meconium aspiration, and increased risk for perinatal mortality. The postterm neonate has a greater risk for respiratory distress, feeding problems, sleeping problems, illnesses, and decreased developmental scores and/or mental scores.

   Maternal consequences of postterm gestation include increased risk for induction of labor and operative birth (episiotomy for macrosomia, use of forceps for macrosomia, and cesarean birth for fetal distress or CPD).

4. Assessment activities during postterm labor include frequent assessment of UC pattern, continuous electronic fetal monitoring of fetal well-being and response to labor, cervical change, fetal presenting part descent, color and character of the amniotic fluid, and maternal and fetal response to oxytocin infusion.

5. Intervention measures for postterm labor include promotion of maternal comfort, fetal well-being (maternal position, oxygen by mask), emotional support, and preparation for operative birth (vaginal or cesarean).

# PROBLEMS WITH THE PLACENTA

**Problems with the placenta** most commonly involve abruptio placentae, placenta previa, or placental insufficiency.

## Problems with Abruptio Placentae

**Problems with abruptio placentae** involve the effect of blood loss on maternal and fetal physiology. The definition, symptoms, consequences, prenatal assessment, and prenatal interventions for abruptio placentae are summarized in the Prenatal Unit (see Chapter 6: "Selected Prenatal Complications").

The cause of abruptio placentae is not known, but it does occur with maternal hypertension (including PIH), sudden decrease in intra- uterine pressure (especially rupture of membranes in an over- distended uterus), trauma, cigarette smoking, short umbilical cord, maternal use of cocaine, and maternal alcohol use.

There are three types of abruptio placentae. Marginal abruption occurs at the edge (periphery) of the placenta and permits obvious escape of blood through the cervix and vagina. The partial abruption with concealed bleeding results in separation at the center of the placenta and traps the blood because the peripheral edges of the placenta remain attached. Blood is absorbed in the uterine muscle (Couvelaire uterus) and causes uterine tenderness and irritability during labor and increased risk of postpartal hemorrhage. The complete abruption is complete separation of the placenta with hemorrhage and fetal demise.

1. Outcome of abruptio placentae depends on the amount of placental separation and blood loss. Cesarean birth is performed for maternal and/or fetal distress. Hysterectomy may be necessary for postpartal hemorrhage due to Couvelaire uterus.

2. Symptoms of abruptio placentae are summarized in Chapter 6: "Selected Prenatal Complications."

3. Consequences of abruptio placentae are summarized in the Prenatal Unit (see Chapter 6: "Selected Prenatal Complications").

4. Assessment activities for abruptio placentae during labor include continuous assessment of UCs and resting tone, continuous electronic fetal monitoring of fetal well-being and response to labor, hourly assessment of maternal abdominal circumference or fundal height, maternal physiological status (vital signs, hydra- tion, color, skin, nailbeds), maternal anxiety level, maternal urine output, amount of blood loss (pad count), color and character of amniotic fluid, and maternal coagulation test results.

5. Intervention measures for abruptio placentae during labor include maintenance of maternal physiological status, promotion of fetal well-being, explanation of abruptio placentae and its consequences, explanation of treatment methods, emotional support,

preparation of mother for vaginal or cesarean birth, and preparation of the unit for vaginal or cesarean birth.

## Problems with Placenta Previa

**Problems with placenta previa** involve the effect of blood loss on maternal and fetal well-being. The definition, symptoms, consequences, prenatal assessment, and prenatal intervention are summarized in the Prenatal Unit (see Chapter 6: "Selected Prenatal Complications").

The cause of placenta previa is not known but it is known to occur in women with previous scars in the uterus (cesarean birth, hysterotomy, D&C), previous placenta previa, multiparity, and increased maternal age.

There are three types of placenta previa. A complete placenta previa is implanted so that the entire cervical os is covered. A partial placenta previa is implanted so that a portion of the cervical os is covered. A low-lying placenta previa is implanted in the lower uterine segment near but not over the cervical os.

1. The outcome of placenta previa is cesarean birth for complete placenta previa or continuous bleeding. Labor and vaginal birth are possible for partial placenta previa or low-lying placenta with minimal bleeding and no maternal or fetal distress.

2. Symptoms of placenta previa are summarized in the Prenatal Unit (see Chapter 6: "Selected Prenatal Complications").

3. Consequences of placenta previa for the fetus include preterm birth, fetal hypoxia, and increased risk of perinatal mortality. Maternal consequences of placenta previa include those summarized in the Prenatal Unit (see Chapter 6: "Selected Prenatal Complications").

4. Assessment activities for placenta previa during labor include those summarized in the Prenatal Unit (see Chapter 6) plus continuous monitoring (palpation) of UCs pattern and resting tone, continuous electronic fetal monitoring of fetal well-being and response to labor, measurement of blood loss (pad count), maternal physiological status (signs of shock), maternal anxiety level, and labor coping strategies.

   NOTE: Vaginal exam on a mother who is bleeding is prohibited. The physician may perform a visual inspection of the cervix using a sterile vaginal speculum in a room with a double set up (set up for vaginal and cesarean birth).

5. Intervention measures for placenta previa during labor include those summarized in the Prenatal Unit (see Chapter 6: "Selected Prenatal Complication") and promotion of maternal physiological well-being, maternal and support person emotional support, information regarding well-being of the fetus, educational preparation

for vaginal or cesarean birth, and preparation of the birthing unit for vaginal or cesarean birth.

## Problems with Placental Insufficiency

**Problems with placental insufficiency** involve decreased utero-placental exchange. Maternal medical disorders (PIH, cardiac disease, diabetes mellitus, hypertension, anemia), smoking, dietary deficiencies, alcohol/drug use, and postterm pregnancy have been associated with placental insufficiency.

The outcome for placental insufficiency can be cesarean birth for fetal distress.

1. Symptoms of placental insufficiency during labor include non-reassuring or potentially ominous FHR patterns and meconium staining of the amniotic fluid (see summary above for fetal distress).

2. Consequences of placental insufficiency for the fetus include intrauterine growth retardation (chronic insufficiency) and fetal distress (acute insufficiency) during labor.

   Maternal outcome is dependent on the cause and also includes increased maternal anxiety levels due to concern for fetal well-being, as well as potential cesarean birth.

3. Assessment activities for placental insufficiency include those summarized above (see Problems with Fetal Distress).

4. Intervention measures for placental insufficiency include those summarized above (see Problems with Fetal Distress).

## PROBLEMS WITH THE PHYSIOLOGY

**Problems with the physiology** involve umbilical cord problems, amniotic fluid problems, and medical disorders.

## Problems with the Umbilical Cord

**Problems with the umbilical cord** most commonly involve cord compression due to cord prolapse, nuchal cord, or oligohydramnios. A rare cause of fetal hemorrhage occurs with rupture of the membranes when there is a velamentous insertion of the cord. The cause of cord prolapse is movement of the cord below the presenting part with the outflow of amniotic fluid when rupture of membranes occurs. Situations at risk for prolapsed cord include unengaged presenting part, small fetus, breech, multiple gestation, extra long cord, low-lying placenta, transverse lie, CPD, or hydramnios. Cord prolapse can be obvious (visible) or occult (beside or just below the presenting part but not visible or palpable in the vagina).

1. Outcome for cord prolapse is cesarean birth for a viable fetus.

**2.** Symptoms of prolapsed cord include the following:
- Rupture of membranes with unengaged presenting part
- Excess amniotic fluid
- Nonreassuring FHR patterns (especially recurrent severe variable decelerations)
- Protrusion of the cord through the introitus

**3.** Consequences of prolapsed cord for the fetus include fetal hypoxia, risk for Central Nervous System damage, and risk for fetal demise.

Maternal consequences of prolapsed cord include increased maternal anxiety regarding fetal well-being and cesarean birth.

**4.** Assessment activities for prolapsed cord include review of maternal history for risk factors, assessment of FHR and FHR patterns following rupture of membranes, vaginal exam for palpation of the cord following rupture of membranes, and continuous electronic monitoring of the fetus with an unengaged presenting part following rupture of membranes.

**5.** Intervention measures for prolapsed cord include relief of cord compression by holding the presenting part off of the cord with two gloved fingers inserted in the vagina and through the cervix, explanation of prolapsed cord and corrective procedure to the mother, oxygen by mask, positioning the mother with head lower than pelvis, preparation of the mother for emergency cesarean birth, and preparation of the unit for emergency cesarean birth. A recommended position for achieving a maternal position of head lower than pelvis is the modified Sim's position with the hips elevated on pillows.

## Problems with the Amniotic Fluid

**Problems with the amniotic fluid** in labor involve the amount of fluid available. Too much fluid (hydramnios) or too little fluid (oligohydramnios) can cause problems during labor. The cause of hydramnios and oligohydramnios are not known. Hydramnios is known to occur with fetal anomalies, diabetes mellitus, and Rh sensitization. Oligohydramnios is known to occur with fetal urinary tract anomalies, intrauterine growth retardation, postterm pregnancy, and early (second trimester) rupture of membranes.

**1.** Symptoms of problems with the amount of amniotic fluid include the following:

**Hydramnios:**
- Fundal height greater than dates
- Overstretching of maternal abdomen (tense, tight)

- Ultrasound data indicating >2000 ml amniotic fluid

**Oligohydramnios:**

- Fundal height less than dates

- Ultrasound data indicating <500 ml amniotic fluid

2. Consequences of problems with amniotic fluid amounts for the fetus include increased risk with hydramnios for fetal anomalies, preterm birth, prolapsed cord, malpresentation, and perinatal mortality.

   Consequences of oligohydramnios for the fetus include increased risk for fetal anomalies (skin and skeletal due to reduced fetal movement, pulmonary hypoplasia due to reduced fetal breathing movements), fetal distress during labor due to cord compression, and emergency cesarean birth for fetal distress.

3. Assessment activities for problems with amniotic fluid amounts include continuous electronic fetal monitoring for fetal well-being and fetal response to labor, careful assessment following rupture of membranes, as well as the usual labor assessments for maternal physiological and emotional status and progression of labor.

4. Intervention measures for problems with amniotic fluid amounts include the usual measures for laboring families, plus education of parents regarding problems with the amniotic fluid amount, and preparation of the unit and family for possible cesarean birth for fetal distress (due to cord compression with oligohydramnios, or malpresentation or prolapsed cord with hydramnios).

   Some institutions treat oligohydramnios with amnioinfusion to prevent cord compression during labor. Nursing assessments and interventions would need to include assessment for effectiveness and adverse reactions to the treatment and parental education for the amnioinfusion procedure.

## Problems with Maternal Medical Disorders

**Problems with maternal medical disorders** due to preexisting disorders and due to pregnancy-induced disorders are summarized in terms of cause/potential cause, outcome, symptoms, consequences, prenatal assessment, and prenatal intervention in the Prenatal Unit (see Chapter 6: "Selected Prenatal Complications"). Extra labor assessments and interventions in terms of those required in addition to the usual labor assessments and interventions and in addition to the assessments and interventions for the specific medical disorder are summarized below:

## 1. Cardiac Disease

a. Additional assessment activities for cardiac disease during labor may include invasive cardiac monitoring for the Class III and Class IV mother and continuous electronic fetal monitoring of fetal well-being and response to labor.

b. Additional intervention measures for cardiac disease during labor include measures to reduce maternal exertion and fatigue, semi-Fowler's or elevated side-lying position (to facilitate cardiac emptying and promote oxygenation), oxygen by mask, medications (diuretics, analgesics, prophylactic antibiotics, digitalis), and instruction in open glottis, pushing with short periods of exertion and complete relaxation between pushes.

## 2. Diabetes Mellitus

a. Additional assessment activities for diabetes mellitus during labor include hourly assessment of maternal blood glucose level to determine insulin need (which is drastically decreased during labor).

b. Additional intervention measures for diabetes mellitus during labor include administration of insulin in an intravenous drip, regulation of the dosage based on hourly blood glucose values, and preparation to discontinue insulin administration during the second stage and early post delivery period when insulin requirements decrease even more than during labor.

## 3. PIH/HELLP Syndrome

a. Additional assessment activities for PIH/HELLP Syndrome during labor include continuous electronic fetal monitoring of fetal well-being and response to labor and medication (Magnesium Sulfate and oxytocin) and assessment for maternal response to Magnesium Sulfate and oxytocin (vital signs, deep tendon reflexes, blood pressure, respirations, urinary output, UC frequency, intensity, duration, and resting time and tone).

b. Additional intervention measures for PIH/HELLP Syndrome during labor may include administration of Magnesium Sulfate to prevent eclampsia, administration of oxytocin for labor induction, avoidance of the lithotomy position (which would intensify risk for fetal hypoxia due to supine hypo- tension), and administration of all intravenous fluids by infusion pump to prevent fluid overload and ensure accurate medication administration.

# PROBLEMS WITH THE MATERNAL PSYCHOLOGY

Problems with maternal psychology involve maternal anxiety levels. Potential cause, outcome, symptoms, consequences, assessment and intervention for anxiety are summarized below.

## Problems with Maternal Anxiety

Problems with maternal anxiety involve the occurrence of excessive maternal anxiety during labor. Physiological and biochemical (including hormonal) changes occur with excessive maternal anxiety. The outcome for excessive maternal anxiety during labor include increased maternal discomfort and potential for prolonged labor.

1. Symptoms of excessive anxiety during labor include:
   **Subjective:**

   • Verbalization of nervousness or no verbalization (too quiet)

   • Multiple questions regarding what is going on or whether or not everything is okay

   • Verbalization of pain inconsistent with objective data

   **Objective:**

   • Noncompliance or too compliant

   • Agitation

   • Tense posture

   • Clenched hands

2. Consequences of excessive maternal anxiety for the fetus include potential for fetal hypoxia due to decreased placental perfusion and prolonged labor.

   Maternal consequences of excessive anxiety during labor include increased labor discomfort and potential for prolonged labor.

3. Assessment for excessive maternal anxiety during labor include assessment of verbal and nonverbal behavior, assessment of maternal vital signs (elevated B/P, tachycardia), and assessment of maternal fatigue level.

4. Interventions for excessive maternal anxiety during labor include prenatal teaching regarding the labor process, education regarding relaxation and breathing techniques, explanation of various strategies for coping with the discomforts of labor, maternal emotional support, and promotion of comfort.

# SELECTED TREATMENT METHODS FOR INTRAPARTAL COMPLICATIONS

Selected treatment methods for intrapartal complications commonly-used for birth due to maternal or fetal distress, due to decreased benefit in continuing the pregnancy, or due to ineffective labor include cesarean birth, induction of labor, and augmentation of labor. Each method is summarized as follows:

## Cesarean Birth

**Cesarean birth** is the delivery of the fetus through an abdominal and uterine incision. Indications for cesarean birth include CPD, failure to progress, severe PIH, active genital herpes simplex, placenta previa, abruptio placentae, transverse lie, breech presentation, fetal distress, prolapsed umbilical cord, hydrocephaly, pelvic contracture, and repeat cesarean birth. The two primary types of cesarean are defined by the location of the uterine incision.

The classical cesarean uses a vertical incision through the body of the uterus. The disadvantage to the classical incision is the risk of uterine rupture with successive pregnancies and the inability of the mother to labor with successive pregnancies (because of the location of the incision in the contractile portion of the uterus).

The lower uterine segment cesarean is the commonly-used type of cesarean. The incision can be vertical or transverse. The lower segment transverse incision is the most common and has the advantages of less blood loss, decreased risk for postoperative infection, reduced risk of uterine rupture with subsequent pregnancies, and permits vaginal birth after cesarean (VBAC) because of the location of the incision in the passive lower uterine segment.

The outcome of cesarean birth is increased chance for maternal and fetal well-being for emergency or medical indications.

1. Symptoms of indications for cesarean birth are included in the summaries of each of the indications included above.

2. Consequences for cesarean birth for the fetus depend on the reason for the cesarean birth and the type of anesthetic administered. Use of general anesthesia increases the risk for neonatal respiratory depression. The most common type of anesthesia for cesarean birth is regional anesthesia (spinal or lumbar epidural).

   Maternal consequences for cesarean birth include disappointment in not being able to achieve the goal of vaginal birth, an increased risk for maternal mortality (due to anesthesia complications or surgery complications), and increased risk for maternal morbidity (infection, embolism, thrombophlebitis).

3. Assessment for cesarean birth includes the assessments for each of the identified indications as identified above.

4. Intervention for cesarean birth include education regarding the indication for the cesarean, explanation of the procedures involved in the cesarean, education regarding the types of anesthesia for cesarean, and emotional support. In addition, if the cesarean is an emergency for fetal distress, information regarding fetal well-being is provided.

## Induction and Augmentation of Labor

**Induction** of labor is initiation of uterine contractions before the spontaneous onset of labor. **Augmentation** of labor is the stimulation or potentiation of existing uterine contractions after the spontaneous onset of labor.

Indications for induction of labor include diabetes mellitus, PIH, postterm pregnancy, intrauterine growth retardation, fetal demise, and premature rupture of membranes. Contraindications for induction include maternal or fetal conditions which would not receive a beneficial maternal/fetal effect from initiation of labor (such as placenta previa, malpresentation, unengaged presenting part, previous classical cesarean birth, CPD, preterm pregnancy, or severe fetal distress).

The primary indication for augmentation of labor is hypotonic uterine dysfunction.

1. Symptoms for induction or augmentation of labor are specific to the above identified indications.

2. Assessment for induction or augmentation of labor include those specific to each of the indications for induction or augmentation. An additional assessment for induction of labor includes assessment of cervical readiness for induction (using Bishop scoring). Cervical readiness can be stimulated using prostaglandin cervical gel.

   The usual method for induction and augmentation of labor is intravenous administration of oxytocin using a piggyback setup and infusion pump and following institutional protocols.

   Adverse outcomes of oxytocin administration include uterine rupture (tetanic UCs), abruptio placentae, fetal distress, maternal soft tissue lacerations, uterine atony and resultant postpartal hemorrhage, and risk for fetal distress due to decreased oxygen supply with hypercontractility, fetal trauma due to rapid birth, and maternal water intoxication.

3. Intervention measures for induction and augmentation of labor include continuous monitoring of UCs, continuous electronic fetal monitoring for fetal well-being and response to UCs, and administration of oxytocin. Other intervention measures include those for each identified indication for induction or augmentation, education regarding the differences between spontaneous labor and oxytocin labor, and emotional support.

# *Unit 3*

## THE POSTPARTAL PERIOD

*The postpartal period, or the puerperium, has traditionally been considered that time from the birth of the neonate until 6 weeks (42 days) past the birth. During the postpartal 6 weeks, maternal physiological systems return to their prepregnant state.*

*Because the postpartal period is a period during which the family makes adjustments to incorporate the new infant into the family and the mother makes numerous physical, psychological, and developmental adjustments, the time frame is often expanded to include the first three months following birth and is called the fourth trimester of the childbearing year. The focus of Unit 3: "The Postpartal Period," will be on maternal physiological and developmental changes, maternal assessment, nursing intervention, and selected postpartal complications.*

CHAPTER 11

# PHYSIOLOGICAL AND DEVELOPMENTAL CHANGES

*Numerous maternal retrogressive physiological and progressive developmental changes occur during the puerperium. Physiological changes are summarized according to organ system and developmental changes are summarized from the maternal perspective.*

## PHYSIOLOGICAL CHANGES OF THE PUERPERIUM

**Physiological changes** are retrogressive (movement backward or return to a previous state) and involve a reversal of the changes of pregnancy. Just as with the physiological changes of pregnancy, the physiological changes of the puerperium affect every maternal body system. Reproductive system, cardiovascular system, respiratory system, gastrointestinal system, renal system, integumentary system, metabolic system, musculoskeletal system, neurologic system, and endocrine system changes are summarized as follows:

### Reproductive System Changes

**Retrogressive reproductive system changes** involve the uterus, cervix, vagina, perineum, ovaries, and breasts. Changes for each organ are summarized as follows:

 1. **The Uterus**

 **Uterine size** reduces at the rate of about 1 centimeter per day after the first 24 hours post delivery. The rapid reduction in size is called involution. The primary mechanism for size reduction is continued uterine contraction. The decline in high estrogen and progesterone levels permit rapid reversal of the uterine size changes caused by hypertrophy and hyperplasia during pregnancy. Hypertrophy changes are reversed by cell atrophy which are enhanced and stimulated by continued uterine contractions.

 Hyperplasia changes are reduced by autolysis of protein material between cells but reduction in number of cells does not occur. Immediately after delivery of the placenta, the uterus is approximately the size of a large grapefruit but gradually enlarges because of uterine relaxation and temporary retention of blood from the placental site. After the first 24 hours it begins decreasing in size on a daily basis until involution is complete.

 **Uterine placental site** changes involve mechanisms to control bleeding. The first mechanism is uterine contraction to constrict blood flow through the uterine vessels. The second mechanism is thrombus formation in the uterine sinuses to prevent blood flow. The third mechanism is exfoliation (sloughing of necrotic tissue) and is the replacement of the thrombus layer with endometrial growth from the edges of the placental area and from beneath the thrombi at the placental site. The process is very similar to the healing of an abrasion on the knee where the "scab" is gradually replaced with new skin from the edges inward and from beneath the scab upward/outward. Exfoliation is necessary to prevent scar formation and loss of an implantation site for a successive pregnancy. Placental site involution is completed by the sixth week (if no complications occur).

**Uterine discharge (lochia)** changes in color and composition as involution progresses. For the first two to three days after delivery, the discharge is red, consists primarily of blood, and is called **lochia rubra**. From about the third to the tenth day postpartum, the discharge is pink to brown, consists primarily of serous exudate, and is called **lochia serosa**. After the tenth day, the discharge becomes a creamy to yellow color, consists primarily of leukocytes, and is called **lochia alba.**

**Uterine shape** becomes globular immediately after delivery of the placenta. It returns to its prepregnant shape as it becomes a pelvic organ again.

**Uterine position** as determined by the location of the fundus is about half way between the symphysis pubis and the umbilicus immediately after delivery of the placenta. The fundus rises as the uterine contractions become less intense and the uterus fills with blood. By one hour following delivery of the placenta, the fundus may have reached the level of the umbilicus where it remains for approximately 24 hours. The fundal height decreases by about one centimeter per day until it becomes a pelvic organ again (by the 9th-10th postpartal day).

**Uterine tone** is very firm immediately following delivery of the placenta. It should remain firm (palpable and contracted) to facilitate involution. If it becomes boggy (soft and difficult to palpate), bleeding is increased and involution is retarded.

Uterine contractions, especially in the multiparous mother, may cause discomfort for the first two to three days following birth. The discomfort is called **afterpains** and is caused by relaxation of uterine muscle cells followed by strong contractions. Oxytocin (such as from breastfeeding) intensifies the afterpains.

2. **The Cervix**
   The cervix gradually closes the internal and external os and returns to its nonpregnant firmness by a week following birth. The external os closes in a slit-like shape rather than returning to its prepregnancy oval shape. Return of cervical mucus production

depends on estrogen and may be delayed in the breastfeeding mother.

3. **The Vagina**
   The vagina gradually loses its edema, regains its pink color, and rugae reappear by about 6 weeks. Return of vaginal mucus production depends on estrogen and may be delayed in the breastfeeding mother until the return of menses.

4. **The Perineum**
   The perineum is edematous and red immediately after birth, especially at the episiotomy site. Ecchymosis may also be present.

5. **The Ovaries**
   Ovarian function returns in the majority of mothers by six months following birth. The nonlactating mother can expect to begin menstrual periods between 6 and 24 weeks. The lactating mother may experience a menstrual period by 30 to 36 weeks. Some lactating mothers do not experience menstrual periods until they have stopped breastfeeding.

6. **The Breasts**
   The breasts have been prepared for lactation during pregnancy. Engorgement (distention, hardness, warmness, tenderness of the breast) is caused by venous and lymphatic congestion. It can occur in the lactating and nonlactating mother (especially if lactation suppression therapy was not prescribed), appears about the third postpartal day, and usually lasts about 1½ days.

   **Colostrum** is a premilk secretion of the breast. It is rich in antibodies, protein, fat-soluble vitamins, and minerals. Breast milk production begins on average about the third postpartal day in the lactating mother.

## Cardiovascular System Changes

**Retrogressive cardiovascular system changes** involve blood volume, cardiac output, blood pressure, pulse, and blood constituents. Changes for the cardiovascular system are summarized as follows:

1. **Blood volume** changes depend on blood loss with the birthing process, movement of extravascular fluid into the circulatory system, and postpartal diuresis. In general, blood volume has returned to its prepregnant level at 3-4 weeks postpartum.

   The increased blood volume of pregnancy permits the mother to lose 300-500 ml of blood at the time of vaginal birth and 700-800 ml at the time of cesarean birth without development of hypovolemic shock.

2. **Cardiac output** increases during the second and third stages of labor and continues elevated for the first couple of days postpartum (due to increased venous return). Cardiac output has returned to prepregnant levels by 3 weeks postpartum.

3. **Blood pressure** usually remains "normal" unless hemorrhage or PIH occur. The mother may experience orthostatic hypotension for a couple of days postpartum.

4. **Pulse** changes are due to the increased cardiac output and increased stroke volume that occur the first week following birth. As a result bradycardia (50-70 bpm) is considered "normal." Maternal pulse returns to the prepregnant state by three months postpartum.

5. **Blood constituents** change postpartally due to excretion of extravascular fluid and reversal of hormone-mediated pregnancy changes.

   a. Hematocrit and hemoglobin levels initially increase during the first 3 days postpartum because of decrease in plasma volume (postpartal diuresis). Hematocrit and hemoglobin levels return to prepregnant levels at 4-5 weeks postpartum.

   b. White blood cell (WBC) count is increased in pregnancy, increases more during labor (due to trauma), and is elevated for almost 2 weeks postpartum. The increase in WBC makes it less reliable for diagnosing postpartal infection.

   c. Coagulation factors are elevated in pregnancy and clotting factors are activated after birth. The activation of clotting factors combined with immobility and/or trauma increase the risk for development of thromboembolism. The coagulation factors return to prepregnant levels a few days after birth.

## Respiratory System Changes

**Retrogressive respiratory system changes** occur rapidly following birth of the baby and delivery of the placenta. Birth of the baby and reduction in size of the uterus remove the mechanical stimulated changes in respiration. Delivery of the placenta eliminates the high levels of hormones that stimulated acid-base balance changes and the hyperventilation of pregnancy.

## Gastrointestinal System Changes

**Retrogressive gastrointestinal system changes** involve appetite, peristalsis, motility, hemorrhoids, and fear of passing the first bowel movement. Each gastrointestinal change is summarized as follows:

1. **Hunger and thirst** are present almost immediately after birth. Use of glucose for the labor process and loss of fluids due to restricted oral intake during labor intensify maternal hunger and thirst. Digestion and absorption (which stopped due to labor)

return after labor ceases. New mothers experience hunger during the early postpartum once needs for rest have been satisfied.

2. **Peristalsis and motility** remain sluggish for a few days due to decreased abdominal and bowel muscle tone and the lingering effects of progesterone and relaxin on the GI system. The mother may experience flatulence the first few days postpartum.

3. **Hemorrhoids** may have appeared due to pushing during the second stage. The discomfort from the hemorrhoids may intensify the mother's fear of having the first bowel movement.

4. **Fear of passing the first bowel movement** because of hemorrhoids and/or trauma to the episiotomy is common. Usually the first bowel movement is passed without discomfort as long as it is not delayed and the stool is soft. Return to prepregnant bowel habits occurs soon after birth.

## Renal System Changes

**Retrogressive renal system changes** involve structural, functional, and fluid changes. Each change is summarized as follows:

1. **Structural changes** include the gradual reversal of the dilation of the renal pelvis and ureter, and the return to the prepregnant tone by six to eight weeks postpartum. Restoration of bladder tone occurs by a week after birth. For the first few days of the puerperium, overdistention of the bladder occurs because trauma to the bladder, transient loss of tone, and residual effects of anesthesia reduce bladder sensitivity to filling.

2. **Functional changes** include the gradual return to normal of the renal plasma flow and glomerular filtration rate by one month after birth. Proteinuria (1+ or less by dipstick) may occur because of the autolysis process during the first week postpartum.

3. **Fluid changes** include marked diuresis that begins by 12 hours postpartum as the extravascular fluid retained during pregnancy is eliminated.

## Integumentary System Changes

**Retrogressive integumentary system changes** involve pigmentation, striae, hair, and sweat gland activity changes. The changes are summarized below:

1. **Pigmentation** changes (chloasma, linea nigra, areolae) regress soon after birth

2. **Striae gravidarum** fade and are reduced in size by 6 months postpartum. In Caucasian mothers, they become a silvery white color and in dark-skinned mothers, they become slightly darker than the mother's skin.

3. **Hair changes** may include increased shedding for 3-4 months and return to prepregnant thickness by 9 months postpartum.

4. **Sweat gland activity** is greatly increased the first 2-3 days postpartum, especially at night. The postpartal diaphoresis assists in elimination of the extravascular fluid collected during pregnancy.

## Metabolic System Changes

**Retrogressive metabolic system changes** of pregnancy that promoted storage and use of nitrogen, fats, carbohydrates, iron, and calcium for fetal growth begin occurring with delivery of the placenta. Return to prepregnant metabolism occurs as soon as hormone levels return to the prepregnant levels.

## Musculoskeletal System Changes

**Retrogressive musculoskeletal system changes** involve collagen and connective tissue, muscle tone, and shift in center of gravity changes. Each change is summarized as follows:

1. **Collagen and connective tissue changes** are reversed by six to eight weeks postpartum. Joint stability is achieved with reversal of the collagen and connective tissue changes.

2. **Muscle tone changes** in terms of abdominal wall and uterine ligament changes gradually return to the almost prepregnant state by 6 weeks postpartum. Diastasis recti (separation of the abdominal rectus muscles) may require a longer time (2-3 months) and abdominal exercises to return to prepregnant tone.

3. **Shift in center of gravity changes** caused by the enlarging uterus are reversed with the birth and involution of the uterus.

## Neurologic System Changes

**Retrogressive neurologic system changes**, such as carpal tunnel syndrome (due to physiologic edema), acroesthesia (due to pregnancy posture), backache (due to shift in center of gravity and pregnancy posture), and faintness (due to postural hypotension), occur after birth of the neonate or within the first week. Maternal headaches postpartum may develop because of PIH or leakage of cerebrospinal fluid into the extradural space (if the mother had spinal anesthesia).

## Endocrine System Changes

**Retrogressive endocrine system changes** involve thyroid, pancreas, pituitary, adrenal, and hormonal changes. The changes are summarized as follows:

1. **Thyroid changes** are difficult to evaluate in the immediate postpartal period because of fluctuation of other hormones. Maternal basal metabolism rate remains elevated for 1-2 weeks postpartum.

2. **Pancreas changes** begin as soon as the placenta is delivered. Diabetogenic changes of pregnancy reverse within the first 24 hours of birth.

3. **Adrenal changes** decrease plasma renin and Angiotensin II levels within 2 hours following birth.

4. **Hormonal changes** include reestablishment of the hypothalamic-pituitary-ovarian function by 6-12 weeks, depending on whether or not the mother breastfeeds. If the mother breastfeeds at least six times per day, her prolactin level remains elevated for more than a year.

# DEVELOPMENTAL CHANGES OF THE PUERPERIUM

**Developmental changes** are progressive (movement forward to a future state) and include phases of maternal adjustment. The phases include the taking-in, taking-hold, and letting-go phases. Each phase is summarized as follows:

1. The **taking-in phase** is a period of passivity and dependence that usually lasts for the first 1-3 days of the puerperium. It is a time of reflection by the mother as she thinks about her new role and relives her birth experience. It is also a time of physical discomfort and energy restoration. The mother prefers and needs for others to take care of her. If maternal physical and emotional needs are met during this time, the mother is ready to move to the next phase.

2. The **taking-hold phase** follows the taking-in phase and is a period of independence in which the mother assumes control over her life. She focuses on caring for herself and her neonate. She is concerned about her bodily functions and is anxious for her body to function "properly." She strives to be the perfect mother and is easily devastated if she perceives her mothering skills are not proficient. She requires emotional support and assistance in setting realistic goals.

3. The **letting-go phase** follows the taking-hold phase and is a phase of interdependence in which the mother and family members develop interactive relationships. The mother gives up her fantasy child and her old role and accepts her real child and her new maternal role. She retains those roles, characteristics, and relationships that are compatible with her role as mother and with inclusion of the child in the family and eliminates those that are not compatible. This phase lasts throughout the child's growing years.

## CHAPTER 12
# MATERNAL ASSESSMENT

*Maternal assessment for the postpartal mother begins with the fourth stage of labor (recovery period) and continues through dismissal from the institution. The first hour postpartum is a critical time period in terms of the danger of postpartal hemorrhage. Careful maternal assessment throughout the first 24 hours postpartum continues to be essential to determine establishment of physiological stability, especially in terms of the ability of the uterus to control blood loss and prevent hemorrhage. The early puerperium is also a critical time for development of the mother-infant relationship and adjustment of the mother-family relationships. Thus, postpartal assessment includes history, physiological assessment, and developmental assessment.*

## HISTORY

The maternal health history includes essential information for identification of risk factors for recovery or postpartal problems and essential information for planning her physiological and developmental adaptation to the role of new mother of one or more children. Physiological risk factors for the puerperium include the following:

- PIH

- Diabetes mellitus

- Cardiac disease

- Abruptio placentae

- Placenta previa

- Precipitous labor

- Prolonged labor

- Cesarean birth

- Retained placenta

Health history components for the fourth stage of labor (recovery period) include pregnancy history, labor and delivery history, and infant history. Additional history components for the remainder of the puerperium include fourth stage of labor history and family profile history.

**1. Health History Components for the Fourth Stage of Labor:**
  **a. Pregnancy history**

- Gravida

- Para
- EDD
- Planned or unplanned pregnancy
- Maternal reaction to quickening
- Completion of the tasks of pregnancy
- Preexisting medical disorders
- Pregnancy induced complications

b. **Labor and delivery history**
- Length of labor
- Fetal presentation and position
- Type of birth
- Use of operative procedures (forceps, vacuum, episiotomy)
- Analgesia
- Anesthesia
- Labor problems (type, treatment, effectiveness of interventions, maternal response)
- Length of time for ruptured membranes

c. **Infant data**
- Apgar score
- Sex
- Weight
- Fetal distress
- Neonatal distress
- Congenital anomalies
- Infant feeding method (breast, bottle)

2. **Additional Health History Components for the Puerperium**
a. **Fourth Stage of Labor/Recovery History**
- Lochia (amount, color)
- Fundal height
- Bladder (empty, filling, full)
- Pulse and B/P
- Voiding (amount, time)

- Perineum (episiotomy, laceration, intact)
- Hemorrhoids
- Breastfeedings
- Mother-infant interaction

b. **Family Profile**

- Number, age, roles of family members in one dwelling
- Type of housing
- Community setting
- Support system
- Educational level
- Occupation
- Socioeconomic status

# PHYSIOLOGICAL ASSESSMENT

**Physiological assessment** begins with the fourth stage of labor and continues on a planned schedule similar to the following:

1. **Recovery Assessment Components** evaluated every 15 minutes for one hour:

- B/P and pulse
- Fundal height (number of centimeters above or below umbilicus)
- Uterine tone (firm, boggy, firm with massage)
- Lochia (amount, color, clots)
- Bladder
- Perineum (episiotomy, intact)
- Comfort level

**NOTE:** Remember to support the uterus with one hand placed above the symphysis pubis when assessing fundal height and tone to prevent inversion of the relaxed uterus.

2. **Transition Assessment Components** evaluated every 30 minutes for one hour and then every hour for two hours (or every hour for 4 hours):

- B/P and pulse
- Fundal height
- Uterine tone

- Lochia
- Bladder
- Perineum
- Comfort level

**NOTE:** The first voiding should occur within the first 4-6 hours after birth to prevent overdistention of the bladder and relaxation of the uterus.

3. **Routine Assessment Components** evaluated every four hours for 24 hours:

- Vital signs
- Fundal height
- Uterine tone
- Lochia
- Bladder
- Voiding
- Perineum
- Breasts
- Heart sounds
- Lung sounds
- CVA tenderness
- Homan's sign
- Mother-infant interaction
- Comfort level
- Fatigue level
- Rest

For the postpartal mother who has completed the first 24 hours with no physiological problems identified, the routine assessment components may then be evaluated every shift, depending on institutional protocol. Assessment data that indicate potential physiological problems include the following:

1. **Vital Signs:**

| | |
|---|---|
| **a.** Temperature | Value >100.4° F. after the first 24 hours (infection; elevation during the first 24 hours is usually due to dehydration) |
| **b.** Pulse | Tachycardia or bradycardia below 50 bpm |

c. B/P        Hypertension (PIH, renal disease, anxiety)
Hypotension (hemorrhage)

2. **Uterus:**
   a. Fundal Height       Elevated or deviated (full bladder, delay in involution)
   b. Tone       Boggy (atony, full bladder, hemorrhage, delayed involution)

3. **Lochia:**
   a. Amount       Heavy (hemorrhage); bright red, continuous flow (laceration)
   b. Clots       Large (hemorrhage)
   c. Odor       Foul (infection)
   d. Color       Failure to progress to serosa or return to rubra (infection, delay in involution)

4. **Episiotomy site**       **(REEDA assessment):**
   a. Redness       Present after 24 hours (infection)
   b. Edema       Pronounced (infection; hematoma)
   c. Ecchymosis       Pronounced (infection; hematoma)
   d. Discharge       Purulent, foul odor (infection)
   e. Approximation       Gaping sutures (infection, hematoma)

5. **Rectum:**
   a. Hemorrhoids       Inflamed, tender (thrombus)

6. **Breasts:**
   a. Color       Reddened area that is painful (infection)
   b. Temperature       Heat (engorgement, infection)
   c. Tone       Hard (engorgement), firm (full)
   d. Nipples       Blisters (incorrect infant attachment), cracks, fissures (risk of infection); inverted (difficult for infant attachment)

7. **Lower Extremities:**
   a. Homan's sign       Positive (thrombophlebitis)
   b. Painful area       Reddened, warmth (thrombophlebitis)
   c. Reflexes       3+ or 4+ (PIH)

8. **Trunk:**
   a. CVA tenderness       Positive (UTI)

**b.** Diastasis recti — Lax muscle tone (pendulous abdomen)

**c.** Cesarean site — REEDA assessment for infection

**d.** Bowel sounds — Absent (paralytic ileus)

**9. Lungs sounds:**

  **a.** Adventitious — Present (infection, airway disease)

**10. Elimination:**

  **a.** Bladder — Distended (urinary retention, risk for infection; risk for uterine atony and subsequent hemorrhage)

  **b.** Bowels — BM delayed for several days (constipation) frequent, loose BMs (diarrhea, excessive administration of stool softeners)

**11. Sleep/Rest:**

  **a.** Sleep — Deprivation (risk for PP "blues," depression)

  **b.** Rest — Interruption (fatigue, delayed recovery)

**12. Comfort:**

  **a.** Episiotomy — Excruciating pain (hematoma)

  **b.** Headache — Excruciating in upright position (CSF leak), with visual disturbance (PIH)

# DEVELOPMENTAL ASSESSMENT

**Developmental assessment** includes assessment of maternal progression through the developmental tasks of the puerperium, and the mother-infant interaction. Developmental assessment is not scheduled as strictly as physiological assessment, but data regarding developmental progression are collected continuously during each contact with the mother.

## Developmental Tasks of the Puerperium

**The developmental tasks of the puerperium** that are observable during the time the family is in the hospital for the birthing process are the taking-in phase and the taking-hold phase. If the mother is a primigravida with an unplanned cesarean birth, she may be in the taking-in phase even at dismissal from the hospital. However, if the mother is a multipara, and the labor and birth occurred with no surprises or complications, she may progress to the taking-hold phase within a few hours of the birth. Maternal progression and observable behaviors may vary based on cultural influences. Assessment for progression through the phases involves documenting the characteristics for each phase.

**1. Characteristics of the taking-in phase:**

- Passivity

- Dependence on others

- Reliving labor and birth experience

- Difficulty in making decisions

- Focus more on self than infant

- Low energy level

**2. Characteristics of the taking-hold phase:**

- Independent

- Increased energy level

- Initiates self-care activities

- Assumes increasing responsibility for neonate's care

- Receptive to education for self-care and infant-care

- Eager to provide infant care "right"

- Easily "loses confidence" in ability to care for infant

- Increased focus on infant

## Mother-Infant Interaction

**Mother-infant interaction** is assessed based on verbal and non-verbal indicators of acceptance of the neonate (bonding behaviors and attachment behaviors) and based on willingness of the mother to provide care for the neonate. Suggested sources of data for acceptance and care are summarized as follows:

**1. Verbal and nonverbal behaviors for acceptance of the neonate:**

- Touching, caressing

- Holding (en-face)

- Eye-to-eye contact

- Talking affectionately to neonate

- Calling neonate by name

- Smiling at neonate

- Identifying family characteristics in infant

- Verbalization of acceptance of neonate's sex and appearance

**2. Neonate care-taking behaviors:**

- Picking up the neonate when (s)he is crying
- Comforting the crying neonate
- Feeding
- Diapering
- Rocking
- Interpreting neonate's cues and behavior
- Asking for information regarding neonate's care
- Asking for the neonate to stay in her room (if possible)
- Verbalizing pleasure with neonate care
- Verbalizing perception of neonate's response to care

Assessment data that indicate potential problems with developmental progression are based on prevention or delay in mother-infant contact or signs of delayed acceptance of the neonate by the mother. Early maternal-infant separation does not mean that a strong mother-infant interaction cannot develop, but it does mean that the "normal" progression is interrupted. In addition, cultural influences may dictate a difference in timing and/or type of behaviors observed by nurses to document achievement or interruption of the progression. Events and situations that can cause early mother-infant separation include the following:

- High-risk labor and birth
- Complication in immediate postpartum period
- Neonatal complication
- Separation of mother and infant

Signs of potential delayed acceptance of the neonate include:

- Refusal to touch or see the neonate
- Delay in naming the neonate
- Delay in maternal care of the neonate
- Negative verbal comments to or about the neonate
- Delayed eye-to-eye contact
- Negative home environment
- Lack of maternal support system

CHAPTER 13

# NURSING INTERVENTION

*Nursing intervention for new mothers involves provision for comfort and physiological well-being; and education for self-care, infant-care, and developmental adjustment. With shorter hospital stays, providing education becomes a challenge to use every teachable moment before discharge. Interventions for alterations in health during the postpartal period are included in Chapter 4: "Selected Postpartal Complications."*

## MATERNAL COMFORT

Provision for **maternal comfort** includes perineal comfort, abdominal comfort, breast engorgement comfort, muscular comfort, rest and sleep. Each comfort intervention is summarized as follows:

1. **Perineal comfort** measures include use of nonpharmacologic and pharmacologic therapy. Nonpharmacologic therapy includes use of ice pack during the first 24 hours, heat (whirlpool bath, sitz bath) beginning 12-24 hours postpartum, and Kegel exercises. In addition, protecting the episiotomy while sitting prevents discomfort. As the mother starts to sit, she contracts her perineal muscle and holds the contraction until she is seated (prevents stretching of the perineal muscles). Pharmacologic therapy includes administration of analgesic medication (usually oral) and/or application of anesthetic sprays PRN.

   Hemorrhoid comfort measures use the same nonpharmacologic and pharmacologic therapy as listed for perineal comfort, plus the use of the side-lying position, Tucks, anesthetic ointment or suppository, stool softeners, and avoiding prolonged sitting.

2. **Abdominal comfort** measures for afterpains include lying in the prone position (stimulates sustained uterine contraction rather than relaxation followed by intense contraction), ambulation, warm bath, and use of analgesic medication. The breastfeeding mother, especially a multipara, will experience increased afterpains with the release of oxytocin with nursing. Administration of a mild analgesic about an hour before nursing will promote comfort during breastfeeding.

3. **Breast engorgement comfort** measures include early initiation of breastfeeding, supportive bra (no elastic straps), warm shower, warm packs or ice packs for the lactating mother.

   Comfort measures for the nonlactating mother include a breast binder or supportive bra, ice packs, and mild analgesic.

4. **Muscular comfort** measures for soreness and aching following the intense work of labor include backrubs, comfortable positioning, warm bath, and mild analgesia.

5. **Rest** measures include providing for periods of uninterrupted rest by organizing care, placing a "mother napping" sign on the mother's door, and transferring telephone calls to the nurses' station while the mother naps.

6. **Sleep** measures include scheduling nighttime maternal assessments during infant feeding times to avoid frequent sleep interruption, assisting the mother in assuming a position of comfort, providing a back rub, and relieving other sources of discomfort (perineal, abdominal, breast).

# PHYSIOLOGICAL WELL-BEING

Provision for **physiological well-being** includes uterine involution, perineal hygiene, breast care, elimination, and nutrition. Each measure is summarized as follows:

1. **Uterine involution** is promoted by maintaining a firm uterus and prevention of uterine atony due to a distended bladder. Reminding the mother to empty her bladder often prevents displacement and relaxation of the uterus. Fundal massage is used to stimulate uterine contraction of an occasionally relaxed uterus. Administration of oxytocin may be required for a persistently atonic uterus (to prevent or halt excessive blood loss).

   Breastfeeding promotes involution by stimulating oxytocin secretion.

2. **Perineal hygiene** measures include changing the perineal pad with each voiding, use of the surgigator with each voiding and bowel movement, and wiping from front to back after voiding or a bowel movement.

3. **Breast care** includes wearing a support bra for the first week for the bottle feeding mother; and a support bra, avoiding the use of soap on the nipples, and keeping the nipples dry for the lactating mother.

   Nonpharmacologic lactation suppression includes the use of a breast binder or snug support bra, avoiding stimulation of the breast, avoiding warm shower water falling directly on the breasts, use of ice packs to prevent/alleviate engorgement, and use of mild analgesia for engorgement discomfort.

   Pharmacologic lactation suppression, when used, involves administration of medications that inhibit secretion of prolactin.

4. **Elimination** measures include reminding the mother to empty Her bladder often even though she may not perceive the sensation of fullness, and administering a stool softener once or twice daily to promote bowel elimination. If bladder distention occurs and the mother is unable to void, catheterization will be necessary.

5. **Nutrition** measures include adequate fluid intake to support lactation and renal function (8-10 glasses of water daily), and a diet which promotes tissue healing (high protein and vitamin C), bowel elimination (dietary fiber), and sufficient calories (complex carbohydrates).

# EDUCATION FOR SELF-CARE

**Education for self-care** includes perineal care, breast care, afterpains, elimination, nutrition, rest, exercise, sexual activity, and immunizations.

1. **Perineal self-care** education includes instructions to change the perineal pad after each voiding or bowel movement, to wipe from front to back after elimination, to apply the perineal pad to the front first (to avoid contamination from the rectal area), and avoidance of tampons until the placental site is healed (cessation of lochial discharge).

2. **Breast self-care** education for the lactating mother includes information about avoiding soap on the nipples (causes drying and cracking), using nonplastic backed breast pads (plastic backing holds moisture in and promotes bacterial growth), wearing a bra to support the heavy breast, and keeping the nipples dry.

   Breast self-care education for the nonlactating mother includes wearing a support bra for one week, avoiding breast stimulation, and completing her lactation suppression medication (if ordered).

3. **Afterpain self-care** education includes information about the cause of afterpains and comfort measures (see comfort measures for afterpains above). Afterpains rarely last past the third postpartal day.

4. **Elimination self-care** education includes fluid intake (8-10 glasses of water per day), roughage in the diet, and perineal hygiene self-care information (see above).

5. **Nutrition self-care** education includes balanced meals that are high in protein and vitamin C to promote tissue healing and contain roughage from fresh fruits and vegetables to prevent constipation.

   Weight reduction dieting during the healing process is self-defeating. For the mother who is obese, a balanced diet based on calories to meet physiologic needs and to meet energy requirements with complex carbohydrates rather than with simple sugars will often achieve gradual weight reduction and promote positive life-long nutrition habits.

6. **Rest self-care** education includes information about resting or napping each morning and afternoon to prevent fatigue, promote recovery, enhance milk production, and decrease the risk of postpartum "blues" due to fatigue/sleep deprivation.

7. **Exercise self-care** education includes gradually resuming daily activities and performing postpartum exercise as instructed by her healthcare provider. Remind her that discomfort or increase in lochia mean that she has been too active and needs to resume activities and exercises more gradually.

8. **Sexual activity self-care** education includes information about using nonsexual intercourse intimacy activities until the episiostomy site and placenta site have healed. The placental site is considered healed when lochia discharge has ceased (about 3 weeks). Episiotomy tenderness may last a little longer if the mother is a primigravida or experienced a 4th degree extension. The vagina is dry because of the decrease in estrogen, and the use of water-soluble lubricant will make intercourse more comfortable for the mother. If the mother is lactating, sexual stimulation will cause leaking. Breastfeeding just before intercourse will reduce the leaking.

9. **Immunizations self-care** education includes information about avoiding a pregnancy for three months following rubella vaccination, and information about the need to administer RhoGam following each birth or abortion (miscarriage) for the Rh negative mother.

# EDUCATION FOR INFANT-CARE

**Education for infant-care** includes providing information and demonstration of daily care activities based on individual parental educational needs. Education can be provided in group classes, one-to- one, by closed circuit TV, and/or videotape presentations. Information parents usually want to know include the following:

- Handling (cradle, upright, football hold)

- Positioning (side-lying after feeding)

- Feeding

- Burping

- Nasal and oral suctioning

- Bathing (sponge bath until cord falls off)

- Tub bathing (baby is slippery)
- Umbilical cord care (keep it dry)
- Signs of umbilical cord infection
- Nail care
- Swaddling/wrapping
- Dressing (1 light layer of clothing more than the parent has)
- Taking the temperature (axillary preferred)
- Voiding
- Stools (consistency, color; number for breastfed infants)
- Diapering
- Sleep
- Activity
- Crying
- Circumcision care
- Safety (car seat, infant CPR)
- Screening tests
- Immunizations

Additional information parents need is a general set of guidelines for when they should call their health care provider for the baby. The following is a general guideline:

- Temperature (100.4° F. axillary or greater; or 97.8° F. axillary or less)
- Frequent vomiting over a period of time (6 hours)
- Loss of appetite (refused 2 successive feedings)
- Blue skin color (especially lips)
- Difficult to awaken (lethargy)
- Apnea (>15 seconds)
- Bleeding or discharge from any opening
- Diarrhea (2 or more green, watery stools)
- Dehydration (<6 wet diapers in 24 hours, sunken anterior fontanelle)
- Continuous high-pitched cry

# EDUCATION FOR DEVELOPMENTAL ADJUSTMENT

**Education for developmental adjustment** includes information about maternal expectations and focus for the taking-hold phase of development and progression into the letting-go phase. Mother and support person(s) need to be reminded that fatigue and sleep deprivation increase the risk for development of postpartal "blues." Suggestions for coping strategies for the first few weeks of adjusting to the new parenting role include the following:

- Set priorities for tasks that need to be performed and identify those that can wait or can be done by others

- Avoid moving to a new location during the puerperium

- Avoid the temptation to perform exceptional housecleaning (identify house cleaning, cooking, laundry tasks that friends or family can perform)

- Schedule naps (at least morning and afternoon the first 1-2 weeks; unplug the phone; do not answer the door)

- Go to bed early

- Avoid accepting any other responsibilities (care of extended family members, community projects, church activities)

- Schedule some quiet time away from the baby and out of the house (family or friends can baby-sit)

- Schedule "couple time" between mother and father

- Select a contraceptive method before the first sexual activity

- Communicate openly with partner and others (share feelings)

- Include the father in the infant care activities

- Plan for infant day care and return to work

- Discuss with partner who will do what activities during the puerperium and after mother returns to work

CHAPTER 14

# SELECTED POSTPARTAL COMPLICATIONS

*Postpartal complications, just as with intrapartal complications, may be expected to occur in the high-risk mother. However, even though most low-risk mothers have no alterations in health during the puerperium, complications can and do occur. The complications can be divided into those that occur during the early puerperium, those that occur later in the puerperium, and those due to preexisting medical disorders or pregnancy induced disorders. Selected compli- cations for each division are summarized below in terms of definition, cause, outcome, symptoms, assessment, and intervention.*

## EARLY PUERPERAL COMPLICATIONS

**Early puerperal complications** are those that occur during the first 24 hours postpartum. The most common early postpartal complication is hemorrhage, which is defined at blood loss greater than 500 ml during the first 24 hours following delivery of the placenta. Early postpartal hemorrhage can be caused by uterine atony, reproductive tract laceration or hematoma, retained placental fragments, uterine inversion, and coagulation abnormality (disseminated intravascular coagulopathy).

1. **Uterine atony** is uterine relaxation/hypotonia. It occurs immediately after delivery of the placenta or within 24 hours of birth and is the primary cause of early postpartal hemorrhage. Uterine atony can be expected in any situation that results in overdistention of the uterine muscle cells or in relaxation or fatigue of the uterine muscle cells.

   Overdistention can occur due to hydramnios, multiple gestation, or macrosomia. Uterine muscle cell relaxation can be caused by administration of general anesthetic agents, administration of tocolytic medications, and grandmultiparity. Uterine muscle fatigue can be caused by administration of oxytocin (induction or augmentation), precipitous labor, dysfunctional uterine contraction patterns, prolonged labor, maternal malnutrition, and maternal anemia. Mechanical factors that can interfere with the ability of the uterus to contract include Couvelaire uterus, fibroid tumors, and full bladder.

   Outcome of uterine atony is increased blood loss. If hemorrhage cannot be stopped by medical intervention, hysterectomy may be performed. Medical intervention may include administration of oxytocics (Pitocin, Methergine) and prostaglandin, fundal massage, bimanual uterine compression, and bilateral iliac artery ligation.

a. Symptoms of uterine atony include the following:

- Relaxed, atonic, flaccid uterus

- Continuous flow of blood from the vagina

- Blood loss in excess of 500 ml

- Symptoms of shock (hypovolemia) occur LATE in the postpartal hemorrhage process. Signs and symptoms of hypovolemia are increasing pulse and respirations, dropping blood pressure, restlessness, and pallor.

b. Consequences of uterine atony include increased morbidity and mortality. Postpartum hemorrhage is one of the leading causes of maternal death.

c. Assessment activities for uterine atony include uterine fundus tone and position, lochia rubra amount and color (bright, dark), bladder distention, and blood pressure and pulse values.

**Note:** Blood pressure and pulse do not reflect the signs of hypovolemia in postpartal hemorrhage due to any of the causes until the blood loss exceeds the amount of circulatory volume increase gained during pregnancy. Then symptoms and consequences of shock progress rapidly.

Since assessment of the degree of saturation of perineal pads does not permit actual measurement of blood loss, perineal pads should be weighed, if postpartal hemorrhage due to any cause is suspected. A general rule of thumb equates a measured weight of 1 gram of blood (weight of a blood filled perineal pad minus the weight of a dry perineal pad) with 1 milliliter of blood loss. Thus, 200 grams (200 ml) plus the average 300 ml blood loss at delivery would satisfy the criteria for postpartal hemorrhage.

d. Intervention measures for uterine atony include careful fundal massage of the atonic fundus (with suprapubic uterine support to prevent uterine inversion) IMMEDIATELY and constant attendance to document maintenance of uterine contraction and amount of vaginal blood loss. If uterine atony returns after fundal massage, the physician is notified and oxytocic medications are administered as ordered and preparation for any additional medical interventions are made. Maternal and family anxiety are reduced by explanation of the cause of the increased blood loss, medical interventions to reduce the loss, and expected results of medical interventions.

**2. Reproductive tract laceration** of the cervix, vagina, perineum, or labia are the second most common cause of early postpartal hemorrhage. Lacerations can be caused by precipitous labor or trauma induced by use of operative procedures (forcep rotation of a posterior fetal position, intrauterine manipulation, midforceps delivery), malposition, shoulder dystocia, compound presentation. Lacerations of the perineum are classified as first degree (skin), second degree (perineal muscle), third degree (through anal sphincter), or fourth degree (through the anal sphincter and rectal wall).

Outcome for repaired reproductive tract lacerations may be increased maternal discomfort, difficulty voiding (periurethral laceration), or hematoma (vaginal trauma, deep vaginal or uterine ligament laceration). Outcome for unrecognized reproductive tract lacerations can be continued, steady bleeding resulting in hemorrhage.

a. Symptoms of hemorrhage due to reproductive tract laceration include the following:

- Firm uterus in the midline at or below the umbilicus

- Steady flow from the vagina, labia, or periurethral area

- Bright red flow is usually indicative of a deep cervical laceration

- Blood loss in excess of 500 ml

- Shock symptoms due to hypovolemia occur LATE

b. Consequences of hemorrhage due to reproductive tract laceration include repair of the laceration (may require a second admission to the delivery area or surgery if the laceration was not discovered at the time of birth), anemia, and blood replacement therapy.

c. Assessment measures for hemorrhage due to reproductive tract laceration include careful assessment of the amount of blood loss, uterine fundal assessment, blood pressure and pulse assessment, and maternal perception of well-being.

d. Intervention measures for hemorrhage due to reproductive tract laceration include explanation of the laceration and repair to the mother, comfort measures (ice pack, heat, analgesia), avoiding insertion of any device into the rectum of a mother with a fourth degree laceration, administration of blood replacement therapy, administration of iron supplement, and promotion of maternal rest.

**3. Reproductive tract hematoma** is a subcutaneous collection of blood beneath intact skin or mucous membrane. It most often occurs beneath vaginal mucosa in the area of the ischial spines and is more common in occiput posterior fetal position, especially if forcep rotation is required. Hematoma can also occur in the area of the episiotomy or beneath the labia.

Outcome depends on the size (amount of blood) of the hematoma. If it is small, reabsorption may be all that is required. If it is large, it will need to be incised and evacuated.

a. Symptoms of reproductive tract hematoma include the following:
   **Subjective:**

   – Verbalization of severe perineal or perianal pain

   – Verbalization of perineal pressure

   **Objective:**

   – Firm, painful perineal area

   – Blue or red discoloration of skin above hematoma

   – Inability/difficulty voiding

   – Firm uterus in the midline at or below the umbilicus

   – Vaginal blood loss less than 500 ml

   – Symptoms of hypovolemia (LATE)

b. Consequences of reproductive tract hematoma may include return to the delivery area for incision and evacuation of the hematoma, increased blood loss, anemia, and blood replacement therapy.

c. Assessment for reproductive tract hematoma includes assessment for subjective and objective symptoms, fundal height and tone, vaginal lochial amount, and ability to void without difficulty.

d. Intervention for reproductive tract hematoma includes reporting assessment findings to the primary healthcare provider, explanation of the cause and treatment for the hematoma to the mother and her support person(s), preparation for treatment, and maternal comfort and hygiene measures.

4. **Retained placental fragments** result in early postpartal hemorrhage by preventing the uterus from contracting firmly to control blood loss. Retained placental fragments can be caused by an extra lobe of the placenta that separates from the rest of the placenta (succenturiate placenta), by massage of the fundus before complete placental separation, or rarely due to placenta accreta (fusion of part or all of the placenta with the myometrium).

Outcome often involves operative removal (curettage) of the placental fragments. Failure to recognize the retention of the fragments can result in early postpartal hemorrhage, late postpartal hemorrhage, and/or infection.

a. Symptoms of early postpartal hemorrhage caused by retained placental fragments include the following:

 - Boggy fundus

 - Increased vaginal bleeding

 - Symptoms of hypovolemia (LATE)

b. Consequences of early postpartal hemorrhage caused by retained placental fragments include increased risk for maternal morbidity and mortality.

c. Assessment activities for early postpartal hemorrhage caused by retained placental fragments include fundal height and tone assessment, vaginal bleeding amount, and blood pressure and pulse assessment.

d. Intervention measures for hemorrhage due to retained placental fragments include reporting assessment findings to the primary healthcare provider, preparation for treatment methods, explanation of the cause and treatment to the mother and her support person(s), and emotional support.

5. **Uterine inversion** was summarized as an intrapartal complication (see Unit 2, Chapter 4: "Selected Intrapartal Complications").

6. **Coagulation abnormality** Disseminated Intravascular Coagulopathy (DIC) is a pathologic disorder which consumes the clotting factors and results in severe hemorrhage due to inadequate amounts of clotting factors. DIC can be caused by PIH/HELLP syndrome, retained dead fetus (fetal demise, missed abortion), abruptio placentae, sepsis, or amniotic fluid embolism.

Outcome for DIC depends on the early recognition of the abnormality and the severity of the blood loss. However, the prognosis for DIC is often poor.

a. Symptoms of coagulation abnormality (DIC) include the following:

 - Spontaneous bleeding from body orifices, gums, venipuncture sites, injection sites

 - Increased vaginal bleeding

 - Petechiae at pressure sites (B/P cuff)

 - Purpura

- Tachycardia

- Diaphoresis

- Hematuria

- Oliguria

- Increased partial thromboplastin time (PTT)

- Prolonged prothrombin time (PT)

- No clot formation for clotting time

- Decreased fibrinogen level

- Decreased platelets

b. Consequences of hemorrhage due to DIC include increased risk for maternal morbidity (renal failure) and mortality, administration of fresh frozen plasma (for clotting factors), and administration of packed RBCs (for anemia).

c. Assessment for hemorrhage due to DIC include review of maternal history for risk factors, assessment for symptoms of DIC, and usual postpartal assessment for fundal tone, fundal height, and vaginal bleeding.

d. Intervention measures for hemorrhage due to DIC include preventing additional trauma (padded side rails, avoiding intramuscular injections, careful placement of the B/P cuff, careful oral hygiene), explanation of the disorder process and treatment regimen to the mother and her support person(s), emotional support, oxygen, intervention for underlying cause of DIC, and promotion of mother-infant relationship.

# LATER PUERPERAL COMPLICATIONS

Later puerperal complications are those that occur between 24 hours and 42 days postpartum. The late puerperal complications can be further categorized according to type of complication. Common late physiological puerperal complications include late postpartum hemorrhage, infection, and thrombophlebitis. Psychological puerperal complications are not common but distinction between the common postpartal "blues" and postpartal psychiatric disorder should be made.

1. **Late postpartum hemorrhage** occurs between 24 hours and 28 days postpartum and is caused by subinvolution of the placental site, retained placental fragments, and/or infection.

Subinvolution is delayed retrogression of the uterus to prepregnant size and function. The most common causes for subinvolution are endometrial infection and retained placental fragments.

Outcome for postpartum hemorrhage due to subinvolution, retained placental fragments, and/or infection include increased risk for morbidity and mortality. It may not occur until the mother has returned home.

a. Symptoms for late postpartum hemorrhage due to subinvolution, retained placental fragments, and/or infection include the following:

- Boggy fundus (first symptom)

- Increase (or cessation of decrease) in fundal height

- Tender uterus

- Increased lochia rubra or leukorrhea

- Backache

- Pelvic discomfort

- Possible foul odor of the lochia

- Anemia (pallor, fatigue, headache)

- Hypotension

- Tachycardia

b. Consequences of late postpartum hemorrhage include treatment with oxytocics, antibiotics, and potential curettage. Blood infusion may be required to correct anemia due to hemorrhage.

c. Assessment activities for late postpartum hemorrhage include assessment for symptoms of late postpartum hemorrhage, fundal height and tone, lochia color and amount, and careful review of maternal history for risk factors.

d. Intervention measures for late postpartum hemorrhage include explanation of the cause and treatment for the hemorrhage, preparation for the treatment methods, promotion of maternal comfort and rest, administration of medications (oxytocics, antibiotics, iron supplementation), and promotion of mother-infant relationship by assisting the mother with infant care (in the mother's room) and ensuring mother-infant visual contact.

2. **Infections** that commonly occur in the late puerperium include UTI, endometritis, and mastitis

a. UTI in the puerperium is often caused by trauma to the base of the bladder and urethra during labor, by intrapartal and/or postpartal catheterization, and urine stasis (due to increased bladder capacity, decreased bladder sensitivity, and postpartal diuresis).

**(1)** Symptoms of postpartal UTI include the following:

**Cystitis:**

- Urination frequency

- Urination urgency

- Dysuria

- Nocturia

- Hematuria

- Suprapubic pain

- Low grade temperature

**Pyelonephritis:**

- Cystitis symptoms

- Chills

- High temperature

- Unilateral or bilateral CVA tenderness

- Nausea and vomiting

**(2)** Consequences of untreated cystitis are progression of the UTI to pyelonephritis. Consequences of untreated pyelonephritis include progression to damage of the renal cortex with resultant kidney function impairment.

**(3)** Assessment activities for UTI include assessment for symptoms of cystitis and pyelonephritis, and careful review of maternal history and puerperal course for risk factors.

**(4)** Intervention measures for UTI include prevention measures (frequent emptying of the bladder during labor to prevent trauma, frequent emptying of the bladder post-partally to prevent overdistention and stasis, increased fluid intake postpartally to promote voiding), careful catheterization intrapartally and postpartally only after other measures to stimulate urination have failed, administration of medications, and educating the mother regarding the importance of completing drug therapy and follow-up care.

b. Endometritis is inflammation of the endometrium. It is also called puerperal infection and was called childbed fever in the past. It is caused by depositing pathogenic bacteria in the cervix during vaginal examination, untreated maternal gonorrhea or chlamydia infection, prolonged rupture of the membranes (chorioamnionitis), prolonged labor, or retained placental fragments. Bacteria migrate to the open placental site and multiply rapidly.

Puerperal infection is defined as a temperature of 100.4° F. on two separate occasions in the first 10 days of the puerperium, excluding the first 24 hours.

**(1)** Symptoms of postpartal endometritis include the following:

**Subjective:**

- Fatigue
- Lethargy
- Lack of appetite
- Perineal pain
- Lower abdominal or pelvic pain
- Nausea and vomiting

**Objective:**

- Temperature (100.4° F. or greater with high spikes)
- Chills
- Uterine tenderness on palpation
- Profuse lochia (or scant if due to beta hemolytic strep)
- Foul smelling lochia (or odorless if due to beta hemolytic strep)
- Tachycardia

**(2)** Consequences of endometritis include increased risk for maternal morbidity and mortality. If untreated, postpartal endometritis can spread to involve the pelvic tissues (parametritis or pelvic cellulitis) and the peritoneal cavity (peritonitis), finally developing into bacteremic septic shock, DIC, and death.

**(3)** Assessment activities for endometritis include assessment for symptoms of endometritis, review of maternal history for prior infections and treatment, intake and output, fundal height and tenderness, and assessment of lochia amount, color, and odor.

**(4)** Intervention measures for endometritis include prevention by using careful aseptic technique, perineal care, careful handwashing, teaching the mother perineal hygiene (wiping from front to back, changing perineal pads with each voiding, replacing the perineal pad front first, sitz baths, surgigator); administration of medications (antibiotics, analgesia); promotion of comfort; and promotion of the mother-infant relationship.

c. **Mastitis** is inflammation of the breast tissue. It usually occurs between two and four weeks postpartum. It is caused by introduction of bacteria into the breast through the nose and throat of the infant or the hands of the mother or nurse. Poor hygiene practices, nipple cracks or fissures, milk stasis, ill-fitting bra, or lack of breast support increase the risk for development of mastitis.

(1) Symptoms of mastitis include the following:

**Subjective:**
- Local breast tenderness
- Malaise
- Headache
- Flu-like symptoms

**Objective:**
- Fever
- Warm area of the breast
- Red area of the breast
- Painful area with palpation

(2) Consequences of mastitis include development of breast abscess, axillary adenopathy, and drainage of the abscess.

(3) Assessment activities for mastitis include assessment of breast color, breast skin temperature, breast consistency, nipple, attachment of the infant to the breast, fit of the bra, and temperature.

(4) Intervention measures for mastitis include teaching infant positioning at the breast to prevent nipple trauma, teaching maternal hygiene methods, teaching support of the breasts (bra with large enough cup to hold all of the breast tissue and no elastic straps), explaining the cause and treatment for mastitis, and reinforcing the importance of completing drug therapy and follow-up evaluation.

3. **Thrombophlebitis** is inflammation of the blood vessel with clot formation. It is caused by the increase of clotting factors and platelets, release of thromboplastin by the decidua and platelets, and increase in fibrinolysis inhibitors.

Risk factors for development of postpartal thrombophlebitis include maternal obesity, increased maternal age, grand multiparity, prolonged immobility (venous stasis), maternal anemia or cardiac disease, varicosities, endometritis, and history of thrombosis.

a. Symptoms of postpartal thrombophlebitis include the following:

**Superficial leg vein thrombophlebitis:**

—  Tenderness along the vein

—  Firmness along the vein

—  Local heat and redness

**Deep leg vein thrombophlebitis:**

—  Positive Homan's sign

—  Pain

—  Temperature

—  Chills

—  Edema

—  Leg may be pale and cool

b. Consequences of postpartal thrombophlebitis include development of an embolism (release of the thrombus from the vessel wall) and the consequences of the embolism (risk of maternal mortality).

c. Assessment activities for postpartal thrombophlebitis include assessment for symptoms of superficial and deep vein thrombophlebitis, review of history for risk factors, and assessment for pulmonary embolism with deep vein thrombophlebitis.

d. Intervention measures for postpartal thrombophlebitis include preventive measures, such as early ambulation, avoiding crossing of the legs, support hose, padding the stirrups (if used), and avoiding the use of the knee gatch on the bed. If bedrest longer than eight hours is ordered, preventive measures include leg, ankle, and foot exercises to promote lower extremity circulation.

Additional intervention measures for superficial leg vein thrombophlebitis include leg elevation, local heat, bedrest, elastic support hose, and analgesics.

Additional intervention measures for deep leg vein thrombophlebitis include promotion of comfort, administration of heparin, preparation for administering the antidote (protamine sulfate) for adverse response to heparin, and administration of antibiotics if temperature is elevated.

For both types of thrombophlebitis, intervention measures also include explanation of the cause and treatment to the mother, teaching preventive measures, and promotion of the mother-infant relationship.

4. **Postpartal psychiatric disorder** includes postpartum depression and postpartum psychosis. To differentiate between the expected postpartum "blues" and the development of postpartum depression or postpartum psychosis, all three are summarized as follows:

   a. **Postpartum "blues"** is a transient, short-term change in affect experienced by the majority of postpartal mothers. It usually occurs between days 3 and 14 of the puerperium.

   (1) Symptoms of postpartum "blues" include the following:

   **Subjective:**

   – Feelings of loneliness
   – Feelings of rejection
   – Feeling "down"
   – Feeling emotional, overwhelmed
   – Confusion
   – Difficulty making decisions
   – Mood swings
   – Fatigue

   **Objective:**

   – Anxious
   – Restlessness
   – Forgetfulness
   – Sleeplessness
   – Exhaustion
   – Tearfulness

   (2) Consequences of postpartum "blues" are usually limited to transient tearful episodes. However, assessment to differentiate "blues" from further development of depression is essential.

   (3) Assessment activities for postpartum "blues" include assessment of maternal/paternal expectations for the puerperium, who will perform what household and infant care activities during the puerperium, support system, maternal coping mechanisms for stress and fatigue, and plans for maternal rest, sleep, and getting out of the house each day.

   (4) Intervention measures for postpartum "blues" include helping the mother and father plan household, infant, and maternal care activities for the puerperium; preparing the parents for the amount of time required in caring for a new

infant and the enormity of the impact on their life-style; and the amount of rest and sleep needed by the mother to recover, lactate, and replenish her energy levels. Intervention also includes suggestions for assistance by support persons and community agencies/services available free or for a fee.

b. **Postpartum depression** includes any of the affective syndromes that occur during the first six months postpartum. The symptoms and episodes of depression often begin about the fourth postpartum week and last longer than the transient episodes of the "blues."

Risk factors for postpartum depression include limited support system, increased stressful life events, limited personal resources for coping with stressful life events (single mother, divorce, separation, recent death of a first-degree relative), and low socioeconomic status.

**(1)** Symptoms of postpartum depression include the following:

**Subjective:**

- Concern about skills to care for infant
- Loss of interest in sex
- Feelings of guilt or worthlessness
- Lack of interest in usual activities
- Fatigue
- Inability to cope
- Change in appetite
- Thoughts of suicide or death
- Insomnia or hypersomnia

**Objective:**

- Weight loss or gain
- Poor concentration
- Difficulty making decisions
- Loss of energy
- Social withdrawal
- Agitation

**(2)** Consequences of postpartum depression include failure of the infant to gain weight as expected and infant irritability.

**(3)** Assessment activities for postpartum depression include monitoring of life stress events, support system, coping strategies for stress, expectations for motherhood, review of maternal history for risk factors, and assessment for symptoms of depression and their duration.

**(4)** Intervention measures for postpartum depression include referral of the mother for professional counseling and/or drug therapy and explanation to the family or support person.

c. **Postpartum psychosis** is severe depression that begins as postpartum "blues" or postpartum depression and progresses to psychosis.

**(1)** Symptoms of postpartum psychosis are usually evident by three months postpartum and include the symptoms of postpartum depression plus one or more of the following:

- Delusions
- Hallucinations
- Confusion
- Delirium
- Panic

**(2)** Consequences of postpartum psychosis include suicide, danger to the infant, and danger to the mother.

**(3)** Assessment activities for postpartum psychosis include monitoring for symptoms.

**(4)** Intervention measures for postpartum psychosis include immediate referral for hospitalization and treatment and explanation of the disorder, consequences, and treatment to the family/support person.

# PREEXISTING MEDICAL DISORDER COMPLICATIONS

**Preexisting medical disorder complications** encountered as early and/or late puerperal complications include cardiac disease and diabetes mellitus. Both disorders are summarized in terms of cause, outcome, symptoms, consequences, prenatal assessment, and prenatal intervention in Unit 1, Chapter 6: "Selected Prenatal Complications." Additional postpartal assessment and interventions are summarized as follows:

1. **Cardiac disease**:
   Assessment activities for cardiac disease during the puerperium include careful assessment for decompensation due to increased venous return to the heart and movement of extravascular fluid into the circulatory system. Postpartal assessment activities also include the usual postpartal assessments for all postpartal mothers for documentation of well-being or early identification of other

complications. The first 48 hours post delivery are the most critical hours for cardiac decompensation.

Intervention for cardiac disease during the puerperium include semi-Fowler's or elevated side-lying position, graduated activity schedule, promotion of mother-infant relationship while avoiding maternal fatigue and exertion, emotional support, explanation of physiological progress and treatment, plus the usual postpartum education and reinforcement of the importance of gradual activity resumption after discharge.

2. **Diabetes mellitus** changes drastically postpartally because of the loss of the diabetogenic effect of the placental hormones. Thus, reestablishment of insulin dosage based on diet and activity (including lactation) is required. Insulin may not be required during the first 24 hours after birth. If the mother is a gestational diabetic, the disease process may be cured by the delivery of the placenta. However, she is at greater risk for development of Type II diabetes mellitus than the average population.

Additional assessment activities for diabetes mellitus postpartum includes careful assessment of blood glucose levels.

Additional intervention for diabetes mellitus postpartum includes administration of insulin based on blood glucose levels, reestablishing insulin dose and diet for glucose control, plus the usual postpartal interventions.

# PREGNANCY-INDUCED COMPLICATIONS

**Pregnancy-induced complications** that may occur for the first time or become worse during the first 48 hours of the puerperium include PIH and HELLP syndrome. Usually PIH and HELLP syndrome improve rapidly following birth. Review definitions, cause, outcome, symptoms, consequences, assessment and interventions in Unit 1, Chapter 6: "Selected Prenatal Complications."

Additional postpartal assessment for PIH and HELLP includes assessment for worsening of the disease process, the occurrence of seizures, and the effectiveness and maternal response to drug therapy (especially overdosing with Magnesium Sulfate as the disease process improves).

Additional postpartal intervention measures for PIH and HELLP syndrome include continuation of medication and promotion of the mother-infant relationship.

# *Unit 4*

## THE NEONATAL PERIOD

*The neonatal period begins with the birth of the neonate and ends when the neonate is 28 days of age. The neonate completes the physiological and developmental transition from intrauterine to extrauterine life during the neonatal period. The focus of Unit 4: "The Neonatal Period" is on physiological and developmental adaptations, neonatal assessment, nursing intervention, and selected neonatal complications.*

# CHAPTER 15

# PHYSIOLOGICAL AND DEVELOPMENTAL ADAPTATIONS

*The physiological adaptations for the neonate from the moment of birth to physiological stability involve every organ system. Developmental adaptations involve progressive daily growth from a dependent fetus to neonatal interaction with people and stimuli within the extrauterine environment.*

## PHYSIOLOGICAL ADAPTATIONS

Physiological adaptations include respiratory, cardiovascular, thermogenic, gastrointestinal, hepatic, renal, immunologic, integumentary, neurologic, reproductive, and skeletal system adaptations. Adaptations for each system are summarized as follows:

1. **Respiratory system adaptations** permit conversion from a fluid-filled system to a system capable of oxygenation.

   **Stimulation** for the first breath includes mechanical, chemical, thermal, and sensory stimuli. Mechanical stimuli are the squeezing of some fluid from the lungs during passage through the birth canal and passive inhalation with birth of the trunk. Chemical stimuli include transitory asphyxia changes (increased $PCO2$, decreased $PO2$, and decreased pH). Short-term asphyxia serves to stimulate the respiratory center, but prolonged asphyxia serves as a respiratory center depressant. Thermal stimuli include the impact of the change in temperature from the warm intrauterine environment to the cooler extrauterine environment. The initial response to the change in temperature stimulates the respiratory center to establish rhythmic respirations but prolonged continued cooling results in depression of the respiratory center. Sensory stimuli include the tactile, visual, and auditory stimuli of the extrauterine environment.

   Once initial respirations are established, the neonate must be capable of producing sufficient **surfactant** (surface tension reducing agent) to reduce the amount of pressure required to prevent the lung alveoli from collapsing with exhalation and to maintain alveolar stability.

   **Respiratory patterns** of the neonate include the following characteristics:

   - Shallow and irregular respirations

   - 30-60 respirations per minute

   - Periodic breathing (periods of apnea for 5-15 seconds)

- Abdominal respirations

- Abdominal and chest movements are synchronous

The neonate is an **obligatory nose breather until three weeks of age. Thus, the nasopharyngeal passage must remain clear to prevent respiratory distress.**

2. **Cardiovascular system adaptations** include transformation from fetal to adult-like circulation. The transformation begins with the first breath and involves closure of the fetal by-passes and changes in pressure.

   **Closure of the fetal by-passes** involves the following:

   a. Foramen ovale closure begins with the inflation of the lungs which causes a decrease in the pulmonary vascular resistance and pulmonary artery pressure followed by a decrease in pressure in the right atrium. The change in pulmonary resistance and pulmonary pressure also increases the pulmonary blood flow to the left atrium which increases the pressure in the left atrium. The pressure in the left atrium is then greater than the pressure in the right atrium and the foramen ovale is functionally closed. A reversal of pressures caused by hypoxia will reopen the foramen ovale.

   b. Ductus arteriosus closure is stimulated by a decrease in prostaglandin supply provided by the placenta and an increase in PO2. Prostaglandin causes ductus arteriosus vasodilation. Increased PO2 causes ductus arteriosus constriction. Thus, the drop in prostaglandin and increase in PO2 result in ductus arteriosus constriction and closure. A decrease in PO2 stimulates ductus arteriosus dilation.

   c. Ductus venosus closure is stimulated by cutting the umbilical cord which causes redistribution of blood.

   **Circulatory pressure changes** at birth facilitate closure of the fetal by-passes and perfusion of body systems. The changes in circulatory system pressure include the following:

   a. Elimination of the placental vascular bed causes an increase in systemic blood pressure and a decrease in venous pressure.

   b. The increase in systemic pressure and decrease in pulmonary artery pressure permits perfusion of body systems.

   **Cardiovascular patterns** for the neonate have the following characteristics:

   - Average heart rate of 120-150 bpm

   - B/P range of 60-80/40-50 mm Hg

- PMI at the 4th intercostal space (visible and palpable)

The **hematopoietic system** variations based on fetal needs include increased RBCs (5.7-5.8 million/cubic mm), hemoglobin (14-29 g/dL), and hematocrit (43%-63%) because of the less efficient oxygen exchange in utero; and the WBC (10,000-30,000 per cubic mm) is elevated because of the trauma of birth. WBC does not necessarily increase with neonatal infection and may instead decrease with neonatal infection. Excess RBCs are lysed in the early neonatal period. RBC life span in the neonate is 80-100 days. **Physiologic anemia of infancy** is caused by the decrease in hemoglobin level during the first 3 months of life.

3. **Thermogenic system adaptations** that permit the neonate to produce heat include increase in basal metabolism rate, muscular activity, and chemical thermogenesis.

    a. The primary means for heat production in the neonate is chemical thermogenesis. The process involves production of heat through rapid lipid metabolism of **brown fat**. Brown fat is unique to the neonate and is located in specific areas of the body. The supply is rapidly depleted during cold stressing of the neonate.

    b. Increase in basal metabolism rate to produce heat requires an increase in oxygen and glycogen consumption. The ill or preterm neonate may not be able to increase oxygen consumption sufficiently for heat production by this mechanism.

    c. Increase in muscular activity (shivering) in response to cold stress is rare in the neonate unless the ambient temperature is below 60° F. It is the last mechanism that becomes operative for heat production and thus is not very effective because brown fat stores have been depleted and basal metabolism rate will have already doubled.

**Heat loss** in the neonate occurs through convection, conduction, evaporation, and radiation.

    a. **Convection** is heat loss from the warm neonate to the cooler air currents (uncovered in air conditioned rooms, unwarmed oxygen).

    b. **Conduction** is heat loss from the warm neonate to a cooler surface in direct contact with the neonate (cold hands, cold exam table, cold scale, cold stethoscope, cold wipes).

    c. **Evaporation** is heat loss from the warm neonate by vaporization of moisture on the body (at birth, during bathing).

    d. **Radiation** is heat loss from the warm neonate to cooler, solid objects near the neonate (windows, outside walls).

**Cold stress** is cooling of the neonate, resulting in excessive heat loss, crying, restlessness, and increased muscular activity which require increased oxygen consumption and energy. Cold stress causes an increase in basal metabolic rate (increased oxygen and glycogen consumption) and, if prolonged, converts to anaerobic glycolysis and resultant metabolic acidosis.

**Hyperthermia** has negative consequences also. The sweat glands in the neonate do not function to reduce his/her temperature. Thus, the overheated neonate can develop cerebral damage from dehydration, or develop heat stroke or death.

The **thermal neutral zone** is the ambient temperature (89.6-93.2° F for the unclothed neonate) at which the neonate is able to maintain the internal body temperature with minimal oxygen consumption and metabolism.

4. **Gastrointestinal system adaptations** include coordination of the suck and swallow reflexes, digestion, and synthesis of vitamin K.

   a. **Reflexes** necessary for feeding in the neonate are the suck and swallow reflexes. Coordination of sucking and swallowing is mediated by neuromuscular maturity which is usually present in the term neonate. A mature gag reflex (present in the term neonate) is necessary to prevent aspiration during regurgitation.

   b. **Digestion** in the neonate is limited during the first few months of life by a lack of pancreatic amylase for converting starch to maltose and minimal pancreatic lipase for digesting fat. Thus, the neonate is able to digest, metabolize, and absorb protein, simple carbohydrates, and some fats. The neonate's stomach capacity is 50-60 ml.

   c. **Vitamin K synthesis** in the intestine requires the presence of bacteria. The gastrointestinal system is sterile at birth. Bacteria are usually present by 24 hours of age.

   **Regurgitation** during the early neonatal period is common because the cardiac sphincter is more immature (in terms of neural control) than the pyloric sphincter.

   **Meconium** is the thick, black, tarry first stool of the neonate. It is composed of contents of the amniotic fluid swallowed during fetal life.

   **Transitional stools** are brown to green stools consisting of meconium and fecal material from breast or formula feedings.

5. **Hepatic system adaptations** include iron storage, carbohydrate metabolism, bilirubin conjugation, and coagulation.

a. **Iron storage** for the neonate depends on the amount stored from the mother in utero and the additional amount stored from lysis of RBCs following birth. The stores in the liver are sufficient to last until about five months of age (if maternal intake was sufficient).

b. **Carbohydrate metabolism** provides the main source of energy during the first four to six hours of life. The neonate's carbohydrate stores (as glycogen in muscle and liver) are low at birth and the relative immaturity of the liver prevents efficient conversion of protein into glucose. Thus, neonatal hypoglycemia in the early neonatal period is common.

c. **Bilirubin conjugation** is the process of converting bilirubin (which is a fat-soluble [essentially insoluble] yellow pigment) into a water-soluble form for excretion from the body. Conjugation occurs in the neonatal liver and requires sufficient liver glycogen stores and enzymes to proceed. Intestinal bacteria convert conjugated bilirubin into urobilinogen which is excreted in the urine and feces.

**Unconjugated or indirect bilirubin** is one of the products of RBC lysis. It moves through the circulatory system by being bound to plasma protein (albumin). In its unconjugated form it can move from the circulatory system to the extravascular tissues causing a yellow discoloration (skin, sclera, mucous membranes) called jaundice.

**Direct bilirubin** is the conjugated, soluble form of bilirubin that is excreted from the liver in the bile into the intestine where it can be further broken down by the bacteria in the bowel into compounds that are excreted in the feces and urine. If there are not enough bacteria in the bowel to convert conjugated bilirubin into compounds excreted in the feces and urine, the conjugated bilirubin is deconjugated back into unconjugated bilirubin and reabsorbed from the bowel into the circulatory system and must be conjugated again.

**Total bilirubin** is the sum of the conjugated bilirubin and the unconjugated bilirubin. When the serum bilirubin level exceeds 20 mg/dL, unconjugated bilirubin moves from the circulatory system into the brain stem and basal ganglia, resulting in **kernicterus** (brain damage usually in the form of cerebral palsy, mental retardation and epilepsy because of destruction of neuronal cells).

d. **Coagulation function** is assumed by the liver during fetal life and to a lesser extent for the first few months of life. The production of coagulation factors by the liver are vitamin K dependent. Thus, until the neonatal GI tract is capable of producing sufficient levels of vitamin K (at about the 5th day of life), the neonate is at risk for hemorrhage.

6. **Renal system adaptations** include function and characteristics.
   a. **Renal system functions** include maintenance of fluid and electrolyte balance. The neonate's extracellular body fluid content is about 40% (as compared to the adult's 20%) which must be maintained. The glomerular filtration rate (GFR) of the neonate is less than the adult and thus decreases the neonate's renal ability to remove nitrogen and other waste products from the blood. In addition, sodium reabsorption and urine concentration is decreased in the neonate. Diarrhea, infection, or feeding problems can result in rapid development of acidosis and fluid imbalance because of the renal immaturity.
   b. **Renal characteristics** of the neonate include the following:
      - First voiding usually within 24 hours of birth
      - Urine color is pale yellow (limited concentration ability)
      - Urine is almost odorless
      - Number of voidings per day of at least 6
      - Limited ability to excrete drugs (renal immaturity)
      - Kidneys are palpable on the posterior abdominal wall
      - Pink-tinged diaper stains are urate crystals (normal)

7. **Immunologic system adaptations** involve active acquired immunity and passive acquired immunity. The neonate's immune system is not activated until about two months of age.
   a. **Active acquired immunity** is the process by which the body develops antibodies specific to illnesses or immunizations. The neonate is able to begin actively forming antibodies at about one to two months of age in response to immunizations or invading antigens.
   b. **Passive acquired immunity** is the passage of antibodies (IgG) from mother to fetus across the placenta and from mother to infant in breast milk. IgG is active against bacterial toxins. Colostrum is high in IgA antibodies that are active in providing protection to secreting surfaces (respiratory and GI tract, eyes).

8. **Integumentary system adaptations** include skin color changes, reversal of birth trauma, desquamation, function of sweat and oil glands, erythema toxicum, and birthmarks.
   a. **Skin color changes** and the cause include the following:
      • Very red (increased concentration of RBCs)
      • Blue (cyanosis due to hypothermia, hypoxia, or both)

- Acrocyanosis (blue feet and hands due to vascular instability, normal for the first 24 hours)

- Blotchy or mottled (possible hypothermia)

- Yellow (jaundice)

- Pink (warm, oxygenated, stable)

b. **Birth trauma** that are common in the cephalic presentation include the following:

  - Caput succedaneum (edema between the scalp and periosteum caused by sustained pressure of the scalp against the cervix)

  - Cephalhematoma (collection of blood between the periosteum and bone caused by pressure of the head against the maternal pelvis; swelling does not cross suture lines)

c. **Desquamation** is peeling of neonatal skin. It occurs with removal of vernix caseosa in the term neonate and is present at birth in the postterm neonate.

d. **Sweat and oil glands** do not function well at birth. Fetal oil glands are hyperactive and produce a protective, white, cheese-like covering for the skin called **vernix caseosa**. **Milia** are distended sebaceous glands that appear as white dots on the neonatal face.

e. **Erythema toxicum** is a temporary, red "newborn" rash that is thought to be an inflammatory reaction that is self-limiting and requires no treatment.

f. **Birthmarks** are skin discolorations noticed at birth. The most common are mongolian spots (blue-gray discoloration on the back and buttocks of Hispanic, Asian, or African descent babies); and telangiectatic nevi or "stork bites" (pink coloration of the nape of the neck, nose, and/or eyelids).

9. **Neurologic system adaptations** include reflex appearance and disappearance which are a reflection of the development of the nervous system. Absence of reflexes that should be present may mean CNS damage and presence of reflexes beyond the time they should cease may indicate CNS problems. Neonatal reflexes commonly present at birth include the following:

- Moro

- Palmar and plantar grasp

- Tonic neck

- Sucking, rooting, swallowing, and extrusion

- Blinking

- Pupillary

- Babinski

- Stepping

- Trunk incurvation

- Wink

- Head lag

- Landau

- Crossed extension

- Arm recoil

10. **Reproductive system adaptations** include pseudomenstruation, swelling of the breast tissue, and descent of male testes.

    a. **Pseudomenstruation** is the appearance of blood-tinged mucous discharge in response to withdrawal of maternal hormones. The neonatal uterus is enlarged at birth due to maternal estrogen and experiences involution early in the neonatal period.

    b. **Breast tissue swelling** is present at birth in term neonates, both male and female, in response to maternal estrogen. Breast bud and areola size increase with gestation.

    c. **Descent of testes** has occurred in the majority of term male neonates.

11. **Skeletal system adaptations** include cephalocaudal development and symmetry.

    a. **Cephalocaudal development** occurs in the direction of head to toe. Thus, the head is larger in relationship to the rest of the body than in the adult.

    b. **Symmetry of size and movement of the extremities** is expected in the neonate.

# DEVELOPMENTAL ADAPTATIONS

Developmental adaptations involve the transition period, sleep-wake cycles, sensory behaviors, behavioral characteristics, and response to environmental stimuli. Each adaptation is summarized as follows:

1. **The transition period** is a period of instability during which the neonate adapts to the extrauterine environment. It usually lasts about 6-8 hours and consists of three phases, the first period of reactivity, sleep phase, and second period of reactivity.

    a. The **first period of reactivity** is approximately the first 30 minutes following birth when the neonate is awake, alert, active, and responsive to environmental stimuli (maternal or paternal voice, touch, breastfeeding). The heart rate and respirations are rapid at this time. The first period of reactivity may be prolonged in an ill or preterm neonate or a neonate that has experienced an abnormal labor process.

    b. The **sleep phase** begins by the third hour of life and lasts from 1-4 hours. During this phase, the neonate's heart and respiratory rate are slow, the neonate is unresponsive to external stimuli, and bowel sounds become audible. The neonate cannot be awakened for breastfeeding.

    c. The **second period of reactivity** occurs sometime between four and eight hours of life. The neonate is awake, alert, and active; often experiences gagging, choking, regurgitation, and passage of meconium; indicates readiness for feeding; and has a higher heart and respiratory rate.

2. **Sleep-wake cycles** occur in the neonate when the period of transition instability has been completed and the neonate is experiencing physiologic stability and behavioral progression. There are two sleep states and four awake states that are summarized as follows:

    a. **Sleep states:**

        **(1)** Deep sleep or quiet sleep behavior includes smooth and regular respiration, no eye movements, and response only to very intense, disturbing stimuli.

        **(2)** Light or REM (rapid eye movement) sleep behavior includes irregular respiration, REM under closed lids, some body movement, and response to internal and external stimuli by smiling or briefly fussing.

    b. **Awake states:**

        **(1)** Drowsy state behavior includes irregular respiration, glazed eyes that open and close, and delayed response to sensory stimuli with smooth movements and possible change in state.

        **(2)** Quiet alert or wide awake state behavior includes regular respirations, bright and wide open eyes, bright facial expression, minimal body activity, and intense focus on environmental stimuli.

        **(3)** Active alert or active awake state behavior includes irregular respiration, less bright open eyes, active body movement, possible fussing, and response increased to disturbing stimuli (hunger, noise, fatigue) by fussing.

**(4)** Crying state behavior includes increased irregularity of respirations, open or tightly closed eyes, very increased motor activity, and extreme response to unpleasant environmental stimuli and internal stimuli.

3. **Sensory behaviors** of the neonate include visual, auditory, tactile, taste, and smell. Neonatal sensory behaviors are present at birth and help the neonate interact socially.

   a. **Visual sense** includes sensitivity to light (frown, blink, pupil constriction), clear visual focus (about 8 inches from the object), and fixation/following of objects.

   b. **Auditory sense** includes the startle or Moro reflex response to loud noise, quieting response to low frequency sounds, and alerting response to high frequency sound, especially the maternal voice.

   c. **Tactile sense** includes quieting response to touch and motion. The neonate is very sensitive to touch and requires it for growth.

   d. **Taste sense** includes ability to differentiate among sweet, sour, tasteless, and bitter substances.

   e. **Smell sense** includes ability of the neonate to recognize the mother by the smell of her milk.

4. **Behavioral characteristics** include consolability, cuddliness, and temperament. Such characteristics are components of the neonate's personality.

   a. **Consolability** is the ability of the neonate to engage in consoling behaviors (hand-to-mouth movements, alerting to voices, cessation of crying in response to voices or touch).

   b. **Cuddliness** is the neonate's response to the body contact of being held (snuggling, molding into the adult's body curves).

   c. **Temperament** is the classification of behavioral style based on activity level, rhythmicity, approach/withdrawal to new stimuli, adaptability, intensity of reaction, threshold of responsiveness, quality of mood, distractibility, and attention span/persistence. The three major temperament categories are the following:

      – Easy (regular body functions, adaptable, positive mood, and moderate sensory threshold and response to new stimuli)

      – Slow-to-warm-up (low activity level, somewhat negative mood, slow adaptability, low intensity of response, and initial withdrawal from new stimuli)

     – Difficult (irregular body functions, intense reactivity, mostly negative mood, resists change/new stimuli, and cries loudly for long periods)

5. **Response to environmental stimuli** include habituation, irritability, and crying.

    a. **Habituation** is the ability of the neonate to reduce physiologic and psychologic response to constant/repetitive stimuli. Habituation is considered protective.

    b. **Irritability** is the degree of crying response (length and loudness) to sensory stimuli.

    c. **Crying** is the method of communication the neonate uses to signal his/her needs (hunger, wet diaper, attention).

## CHAPTER 16
# NEONATAL ASSESSMENT

*Neonatal assessment begins at the moment of birth with the Agpar scoring and initial assessment of physiological well-being. After the neonate is physiologically stable (and by 4-8 hours of age), a thorough physical assessment and gestational age assessment are completed.*

## PHYSICAL ASSESSMENT

The neonatal physical assessment begins with a review of history and concludes with a head-to-toe physical assessment. Components of the history and assessment are summarized as follows:

### History Components

History components to be reviewed in assessing neonatal well-being and planning for neonatal care include the following:

- Maternal prenatal history

- Maternal labor and birth history

- Fetal response to the birthing process

- Maternal medications during the birthing process

- Apgar score values at 1 and 5 minutes

- Neonatal treatments at the time of birth

### Physical Assessment Components

The neonatal physical assessment proceeds from head-to-toe and includes the following components and expected findings:

| COMPONENT | EXPECTED FINDINGS |
| --- | --- |
| Posture (at rest) | Flexed extremities, clenched fists |
| Body/Muscle Tone | Resists extension of extremities (assessed throughout) |
| Moro Reflex | Response to loud sound, loss of support |
| Vital Signs | |
| Temperature | 97-99° F axillary |

| COMPONENT *(Cont'd.)* | EXPECTED FINDINGS *(Cont'd.)* |
|---|---|
| Heart rate | 120-160 bpm (at rest)<br>160-180 bpm (crying)<br>80-120 bpm (deep sleep) |
| Respiratory rate | 30-60 rpm<br>>60 rpm (crying) |
| **Vital Statistics** | |
| Weight | 2500-4000 grams (5lb 8oz -<br>8lb 13oz)<br><2748 grams (SGA or preterm)<br>>4000 grams (LGA) |
| Length | 18-22 inches (45-55 cm) |
| Head circumference | 12.5-14.5 inches (32-37 cm) |
| Chest circumference | 2 cm less than head circumference |
| Abdominal circumference | Approximately the same as chest |
| **Skin** | |
| Color | Pink or consistent with ethnicity |
| Lanugo | Amount (decreases with gestational age) |
| Turgor | Elastic |
| **Head** | |
| Molding | Overlapping suture lines present |
| Anterior fontanelle | Diamond shape (3-4cm × 2-3cm)<br>Depressed in dehydration<br>Bulging in intracranial pressure |
| Posterior fontanelle | Triangle shape (0.5-1.0cm) |
| Hair | Fine, color |
| Face | Symmetry of features and movement<br>Eyebrows and eyelashes present |
| Eyes | Blue, slate gray<br>White sclera<br>PERRLA, red reflex, blink reflex |
| Mouth | Epstein's pearls<br>Intact hard and soft palate<br>Uvula midline<br>Root, suck, swallow, gag, extrusion reflexes |
| Nose | Nares patent (obligatory nose breather) |

| COMPONENT *(Cont'd.)* | EXPECTED FINDINGS *(Cont'd.)* |
|---|---|
| Milia | Present on face (bridge of nose, chin) |
| Ears | Symmetric<br>Top in line with eye canthi<br>Hearing (responds to sounds) |
| Head lag | 45 ° or less |
| **Neck** | |
| Mobility | Full range of motion |
| Thyroid gland | Nonpalpable |
| Lymph nodes | Nonpalpable |
| Clavicles | Intact |
| Control | Raises head when prone<br>Brief control in erect position |
| Reflex | Tonic neck |
| **Chest** | |
| Shape | Cylindric, symmetric |
| Expansion abdomen | Symmetric; synchronous with |
| Auscultation Auscultation) | Lung sounds CTA (Clear to<br><br>Heart sounds rate, regularity, rhythm |
| PMI interspace | Palpable & observable at 4th |
| Breast | Palpable bud (5-10mm) |
| Brachial pulses | Palpable, equal bilaterally<br>Equal with PMI |
| **Abdomen** | |
| Shape | Round, symmetric |
| Umbilicus | 2 arteries, 1 vein<br>No protrusion |
| Auscultation | Bowel sounds present @ 1-2 hours of life |
| Palpation | Slight diastasis recti<br>Liver edge (@-1cm below costal margin)<br>Spleen (@ left costal margin)<br>Kidneys |
| Percussion | Liver, spleen size |

| Component *(Cont'd)* | Expected Findings *(Cont'd )* |
|---|---|
| Femoral pulses | Palpable equal bilaterally<br>Equal with PMI |
| **Genitalia** | |
| Urination | First voiding within 24 hours of age |
| **Labia** | **Majora > or cover minora** |
| Vagina | Vaginal tag<br>Mucous and/or bloody discharge |
| Penis | Meatus at tip<br>Foreskin adherent to glans |
| Scrotum | Rugae, testes descended |
| **Back and Anus** | |
| Buttocks | Symmetrical |
| Spine | Straight, flexible |
| Alignment | Shoulders, scapulae, & iliac crests |
| Sacrum | intact |
| Reflexes<br>extension, | Trunk incurvation, crossed<br><br>Landau |
| Anus | Patent<br>Meconium, transitional stools<br>Wink reflex |
| **Extremities** | |
| Arms | Symmetry of movement<br>Flexed at rest<br>Equal length<br>Moro reflex response<br>Palmar grasp |
| Hands | Fingers separate, 5 each hand<br>Finger nails present<br>Palmar crease normal |
| Legs | Symmetry of movement<br>Flexed at rest<br>Equal length, symmetric skin folds<br>Ortolani maneuver (no dislocation or clicks)<br>Stepping reflex |
| Feet | Plantar sole creases<br>5 separate toes each foot<br>Plantar grasp<br>Babinski reflex |

# GESTATIONAL AGE ASSESSMENT

Gestational age assessment is completed ideally by four hours of age. The scoring to determine age within a few hours of birth is based on a modified version of the Dubowitz assessment tool and is called the Ballard Scale. Once gestation age is determined, the neonate is then classified in terms of appropriateness of size for gestational age. Gestational age assessment and size appropriateness determination are essential for early identification of alterations due to age or size and planning intervention for the alterations.

## Ballard Scale Assessment of Gestational Age

The **Ballard Scale** assessment of gestational age consists of a neuromuscular maturity portion and a physical maturity portion. Each portion of the scale has 6 assessment components which are scored based on specific criteria for each component. A summary of the components, score value, and criteria are summarized as follows:

1. **Neuromuscular Maturity** (based on flexibility and resistance):

| ASSESSMENT COMPONENT | VALUE | CRITERIA |
|---|---|---|
| a. Posture at rest | 0 | Extension of all extremities |
| | 1 | Extension of arms Beginning flexion of thighs |
| | 2 | Extension of arms Beginning flexion of legs |
| | 3 | Beginning flexion of arms, flexion of legs |
| | 4 | Complete flexion of arms and legs |
| b. Square window | 0 | 90° angle (Hypothenar eminence & forearm) |
| | 1 | 60° angle |
| | 2 | 45° angle |
| | 3 | 30° angle |
| | 4 | 0° angle |
| c. Arm recoil | 0 | Arms remain extended |
| | 1 | 140°-180° angle (at elbow) |

| ASSESSMENT COMPONENT | VALUE | CRITERIA |
|---|---|---|
| c. Arm recoil (cont'd) | 2 | 110°-140° angle |
| | 3 | 90°-100° angle |
| | 4 | <90° angle |
| d. Popliteal angle | 0 | 160° angle (extension) (angle behind the knee) |
| | 1 | 140° angle |
| | 2 | 120° angle |
| | 3 | 100° angle |
| | 4 | 90° angle |
| | 5 | <90° angle |
| e. Scarf sign | 0 | Elbow at opposite shoulder |
| | 1 | Elbow at opposite nipple |
| | 2 | Elbow at midline |
| | 3 | Elbow at same side nipple |
| | 4 | Elbow at same side shoulder |
| f. Heel to ear | 0 | Toes touch ear, 180° angle (behind knee) |
| | 1 | Toes almost touch face, 130° angle |
| | 2 | 110° angle |
| | 3 | 90° angle |
| | 4 | <90° angle |
| 2. Physical Maturity: | | |
| a. Skin | 0 | Edematous extremities, color red, skin transluscent |
| | 1 | Smooth pink color, visible veins |
| | 2 | No edema, superficial peeling and/or rash, few veins |
| | 3 | Cracking, pale areas, rare veins |

| ASSESSMENT COMPONENT | VALUE | CRITERIA |
|---|---|---|
| a. Skin (cont'd) | 4 | Deep cracking, parchment-like skin, no veins |
| | 5 | Cracked, wrinkled, leathery |
| b. Lanugo | 0 | Sparse |
| | 1 | Abundant |
| | 2 | Thinning |
| | 3 | Bald areas |
| | 4 | Mostly bald |
| c. Plantar creases | 0 | None |
| | 1 | Faint red marks (upper ½ sole) |
| | 2 | Anterior transverse crease only |
| | 3 | Creases over anterior ⅔ of sole |
| | 4 | Creases cover entire sole |
| d. Breast | 0 | Nipple barely perceptible, no palpable breast bud |
| | 1 | Nipple present, flat areola, no palpable breast bud |
| | 2 | Stippled areola with flat edge, 1-2mm breast bud |
| | 3 | Raised areola with raised edge, 3-4mm breast bud |
| | 4 | Full areola & 5-10mm breast bud |
| e. Eye/Ear | 0 | Lids open, Pinna flat (no cartilage), soft remains folded |

| ASSESSMENT COMPONENT | VALUE | CRITERIA |
|---|---|---|
| e. Eye/Ear (cont'd) | 1 | Slightly curved pinna, soft slow recoil (unfolding) |
| | 2 | Well-curved pinna, soft ready recoil |
| | 3 | Formed pinna, firm to edge<br>Instant recoil |
| | 4 | Thick cartilage, ear stiff |
| f. Genitals | | |
| Male: | 0 | No testes in scrotum, faint rugae present |
| | 1 | Testes in upper canal |
| | 2 | Testes descending, rare rugae |
| | 3 | Testes within scrotum, good rugae |
| | 4 | Testes in pendulous scrotum, deep rugae |
| Female: | 0 | Prominent clitoris & small labia minora |
| | 1 | Prominent clitoris & enlarging labia minora |
| | 2 | Labia majora & minora equally prominent |
| | 3 | Labia majora appear large, labia minora appear small |
| | 4 | Labia majora completely cover labia minora & clitoris |

TOTAL SCORE: ____

3. **Maturity Rating** is determined by comparing the total score with the corresponding weeks gestation according to the following values:

| TOTAL SCORE | WEEKS GESTATION |
|---|---|
| 0 | 24 |
| 5 | 26 |
| 10 | 28 |

| TOTAL SCORE *(Cont'd.)* | WEEKS GESTATION *(Cont'd.)* |
|---|---|
| 15 | 30 |
| 20 | 32 |
| 25 | 34 |
| 30 | 36 |
| 35 | 38 |
| 40 | 40 |
| 45 | 42 |
| 50 | 44 |

# Classification of Appropriateness of Size for Age

**Classification of appropriateness of size for age** is based on the neonate's weight for each week of gestation. There are three classes of the classification. Each class is summarized as follows:

1 **Small for gestational age** (SGA) is a neonate whose weight is below the 10th percentile for his/her weeks of gestation.

2. **Appropriate for gestational age** (AGA) is a neonate whose weight is between the 10th and 90th percentiles for his/her weeks of gestation.

3. **Large for gestational age** (LGA) is a neonate whose weight is above the 90th percentile for his/her weeks of gestation.

# Other Neonatal Classifications

**Other neonatal classifications** for neonates are based on the gestational age or size. Each classification is summarized below:

1. **Classification according to gestational age:**

   a. **Preterm/Premature** is a neonate whose gestational age is 37 weeks or less.

   b. **Term** is a neonate whose gestational age is 38-42 weeks.

   c. **Postterm/Postmature** is a neonate whose gestational age is more than 42 weeks.

2. **Classification according to size:**

   a. **Low birth weight** (LBW) is a neonate whose birth weight is 2500 grams or less. The LBW neonate may be term, preterm, or postterm.

   b. **Intrauterine growth retardation** (IUGR) is a neonate whose intrauterine rate of growth did not meet expected values. The IUGR neonate may be term, preterm, or postterm.

   Classification according to size alone does not provide as much information as classification according to gestational age and size (weight).

# CHAPTER 17
# NURSING INTERVENTION

*Nursing intervention for term, well neonates can be divided into three phases, admission intervention, on-going intervention, and discharge intervention. Admission intervention is the most intense because of the physiological instability of the neonate and because of the tasks involved in admission. On-going intervention is less intense and more maintenance oriented. Preparation for discharge interventions focus on preparation for family functioning during the remainder of the neonatal period.*

## ADMISSION INTERVENTION

**Admission intervention** involves activities to facilitate neonatal progression through the transition phase and establishment of a foundation for maintenance of stability. The intervention activities include establishing a clear airway, a neutral thermal environment, hygiene, preventing hemorrhage, eye prophylaxis, initiating the first feeding, and promoting parent-infant interaction.

1. **Establishing a clear airway** activities include suctioning mucus from the nasal and oral passages, positioning the neonate in the side-lying position, and careful observation. If wall suction is used to remove mucus from the stomach, care must be taken to avoid stimulation of the vagus nerve with insertion of the catheter resulting in bradycardia and hypoxia at a critical physiological time.

2. **Establishing a neutral thermal environment** activities include preheating the radiant warmer before birth, quickly drying the amniotic fluid from the neonate at birth, placing the neonate on a warm and dry surface (mother's skin or radiant warmer), and providing a source of heat over the neonate (radiant warmer over neonate or neonate/mother and neonate or warmed blankets over mother and neonate).

3. **Hygiene** intervention begins with the admission bath. The bath can be given after parents and neonate have had time to interact and the neonate's temperature is at least 97.7° F axillary. The bath is given in the radiant warmer (usually in the mother's LDR or LDRP room) to prevent cold stressing the neonate. The admission bath includes a shampoo. The neonate's temperature is reassessed after the bath. With a temperature of at least 97.7° F, the neonate can be dressed, wrapped in double blankets, a stockinette cap placed on his/her head, and placed in an open crib. The temperature is assessed often the first 4 hours after the bath to identify cold stressing early.

4. **Preventing hemorrhage** activity includes prophylactic injection of vitamin K (since the infant does not produce his/her own vitamin K in the intestine yet). The injection should be given after the bath to prevent providing a portal of entry for organisms on the neonatal skin from the amniotic fluid. The injection is given in the vastus lateralis muscle of the thigh.

5. **Eye prophylaxis** activity is a legal requirement to prevent ophthalmia neonatorum from organisms which could be present in the birth canal. The usual medication is erythromycin ophthalmic ointment which is placed in a narrow ribbon from the inner canthus to the outer canthus along the conjunctiva of the lower lid on each eye. Since the ointment interferes with eye-to-eye contact between parent and infant, administration can be delayed until after the initial parent-infant contact of the first reactive phase as long as it is administered by 2 hours of age.

6. **Initiating the first feeding** for the breastfeeding neonate needs to occur ideally during the first reactive phase (first 30 minutes after birth). If the breast-feeding or bottle-feeding neonate's glucose level is within the euglycemic range, the first feeding may not occur until the second reactive phase. The neonate signals readiness for feeding by crying, exhibiting sucking and rooting behaviors, and has active bowel sounds.

7. **Promoting parent-neonate interaction** activities during the transition phase include positioning the neonate for parent and neonate eye-to-eye contact (about eight inches face-to-face), encouraging parental touch, role-modeling calling the neonate by name (or at least asking about the neonate's name), identifying positive physical characteristics of the neonate, and helping the parents identify family characteristics in the neonate. Separating the parents and neonate during the first reactive phase for nursing admission interventions does NOT promote parent- neonate interaction.

# ON-GOING INTERVENTION

**On-going intervention** involves activities for maintenance of neonatal physiological stability and progressive neonate-parent relationship development. On-going activities include maintaining a protective environment, maintaining physiological functions, maintaining hygiene, promoting safety, promoting parent-neonate interaction, and providing therapeutic interventions.

1. **Maintaining a protective environment** activities include complying with the CDC Universal Precautions for Body Fluids, good handwashing technique (the MOST important protective activity), and exclusion of personnel with infectious disorders from providing neonatal care.

2. **Maintaining physiological functions** activities include the following:

a. Prevent cold stress by providing a neutral thermal environment (70° F ambient room temperature for dressed and wrapped neonate), reducing the time the neonate is undressed, or placing the neonate in the radiant warmer if prolonged periods without clothes are required for procedures. If hypothermia does occur, the neonate must be gradually rewarmed to prevent apnea and acidosis.

b. Enhance adequate oxygenation by maintaining a clear airway, suctioning excess mucus from the oral and nasal passages as it occurs (remember to compress the bulb syringe before insertion), relieving airway obstruction when choking occurs (back blows), and positioning the neonate in a side-lying position with a blanket roll support so that oral fluid can drain out the side of the mouth.

c. Ensure adequate nutrition by providing education and emotional support for the mother's selected method of feeding her neonate. Neonatal nutritional needs include the following:

(1) 50-55 calories/lb/day (105-110 calories/kg/day);

(2) 64-73 ml fluid/lb/day (140-160 ml fluid/kg/day);

(3) Carbohydrate (50%-55% of calories);

(4) Easily digestible fat (30%-35% of calories); and

(5) Protein (2.2g/kg/day)

The initial feeding for bottle fed neonates in many institutions is sterile water. The rationale is that sterile water can be absorbed from the lung should aspiration occur due to uncoordinated suck and swallow reflexes or esophageal abnormalities. The initial feeding usually occurs at least by 4 hours of age. Colostrum is nonirritating if aspirated.

Educational preparation of the parents for bottle feeding includes teaching the following:

– Positioning of the neonate

– Holding the bottle

– Burping technique and frequency

– Eye-to-eye contact

– Bottle and nipple preparation

– Formula preparation

– Formula storage

– Neonatal hunger behavior

– Neonatal satiation behavior

Educational preparation of the parents for breastfeeding include the following:

- – Positioning of the neonate
- – Supporting the breast
- – Burping technique and frequency
- – Eye-to-eye contact
- – Breast care
- – Let-down reflex
- – Removing the neonate from the breast
- – Maternal dietary and fluid intake
- – Growth spurts
- – Milk production (demand and supply)
- – Expression of milk
- – Storing of milk
- – Emotional support
- – Neonatal hunger behavior
- – Frequency of feedings
- – Neonatal satiation behavior
- – Determining adequacy of feeding (6 wet diapers/day)
- – Breast milk stools

   d. Respond to crying cue by talking to the neonate, determine the cause of the discomfort signaled by the crying, correct the cause, pick up the neonate, cuddle and console the neonate.

3. **Maintaining hygiene** activities include providing/teaching cord care, diaper changing and perineal cleansing, bathing (sponge bath until cord falls off and site is healed), wrapping, and dressing the neonate. Nursing intervention also includes maintaining clean linens in the neonate's crib.

4. **Promoting safety** activities include demonstrating/teaching holding, positioning, burping, temperature assessment, and suctioning of the neonate.

5. **Promoting neonate and parent interaction** activities include providing opportunities for parents to be involved in their neonate's care in a supportive environment. Frequent contact is provided by rooming-in, mother-baby care, LDR (Labor, Delivery, and Recovery in the same room), and LDRP (Labor, Delivery, Recovery, and Postpartum in the same room) arrangements in the perinatal unit.

6. **Providing therapeutic interventions** include the following:

    a. Phototherapy for physiologic jaundice or hyperbilirubinemia uses fluorescent bulbs to convert unconjugated bilirubin into components that are excreted in the urine and stool. Intervention activities for phototherapy include the following:

        **(1)** Exposure of as much skin surface as possible (unclothed except for diaper);

        **(2)** Protection of the retina by use of eye patches which are removed for eye-to-eye contact during feedings and eye assessment;

        **(3)** Prevention of hyperthermia and hypothermia;

        **(4)** Prevention of dehydration;

        **(5)** Prevention of diaper rash due to frequent, loose stools;

        **(6)** Promotion of parent and neonate contact (phototherapy in mother's room, home phototherapy, parental nursery visits).

    b. Circumcision methods include the Plastibell or the Yellen clamp technique. Nursing intervention includes educational preparation of the parents regarding the procedure and care of the neonate following the procedure, monitoring the neonate for hemorrhage and voiding, and neonatal comfort measures.

    c. Collections of specimens from the neonate commonly involve heel stick for glucose level, newborn screening, and bilirubin level. Care must be exercised to avoid nerves and arteries in the heel and to prevent scar formation on the bottom of the foot. The usual site for the heel stick is the outer, lateral edge of the heel.

# DISCHARGE INTERVENTION

**Discharge intervention** involves activities to prepare the family to maintain neonatal physiological stability and promote family relationship development. Intervention activities for discharge include the following:

1. **Monitoring parental knowledge and skills** for maintaining physiological stability such as the following:

    a. Body temperature (clothing, taking temperature);

    b. Respiration (sneezing to clear air passages, maternal URI, cigarette smoking pollution, suffocation, aspiration, symptoms of the common cold);

    **c.** Elimination (stools, voidings, number, color, odor, consistency);

    **d.** Safety (car restraint, supervising sibling-neonatal contact, sharp objects, small objects, rolling off surfaces);

    **e.** Immunizations; and

    **f.** Infant follow-up care.

2. **Providing parental education** intervention includes educational needs identification by the individual parents and usually includes areas such as those itemized in the Postpartal Unit, Chapter 3, "Nursing Intervention."

3. **Promoting family relationship development** activities include anticipatory guidance for the first weeks at home, parental fatigue levels, neonate's unique personality, planning activities, and establishing realistic expectations (see Unit 3, Chapter 3, "Nursing Intervention").

CHAPTER 18

# SELECTED NEONATAL COMPLICATIONS

*Neonatal complications can occur in high-risk or low-risk neonates. However, neonates born to mothers with high-risk pregnancies or birthing processes tend to experience more complications. The selected neonatal complications presented are divided into those due to age and size classification, those due to physiological problems, and those due to acquired problems. Each complication is summarized as to definition, cause, outcome, physiological problems or symptoms, consequence, assessment, and intervention.*

## AGE AND SIZE CLASSIFICATION PROBLEMS

**Age and size classification problems** involve the SGA, LGA, preterm, and postterm neonate. Each is summarized below.

   1. **SGA** (Small for Gestational Age) neonates are smaller than expected for their gestational age; i.e., preterm SGA, term SGA, postterm SGA. SGA is caused by intrauterine growth retardation (IUGR). IUGR can occur at any time during pregnancy. If it occurs in early pregnancy and continues, the neonate experiences symmetric (decrease in cell number) IUGR and is small in length, head circumference, and weight. If IUGR occurs in the latter part of pregnancy, the neonate experiences asymmetric (decrease in cell size) IUGR and is small primarily in weight (length and head circumference are above the 10th percentile).

   Causes of symmetric IUGR include infections, chronic hypertension, chronic intrauterine infection, substance abuse, anemia, severe malnutrition, teratogens, and chromosomal abnormalities. Causes of asymmetric IUGR include maternal and placental factors. Maternal factors are any cause of inadequate weight gain, such as lack of prenatal care, age (<16 or >40), smoking, low socioeconomic status, closely spaced pregnancies (grand multiparity), heart disease, substance abuse, sickle cell anemia, asymptomatic pyelonephritis, undernutrition, anemia, and conditions which cause interference with placental perfusion (PIH and advanced diabetes mellitus). Placental factors include any cause of interference with placental exchange (infarcts, cord anomalies, and placenta previa).

   Outcome for symmetric IUGR can be poor brain development due to impact of IUGR on all organ systems. Outcome for asymmetric IUGR can include various learning difficulties. Asymmetric IUGR neonates tend to "catch up" with age mates in terms of size but symmetric IUGR neonates tend to remain small.

a. Common physiologic problems of the SGA neonate include the following:

- Perinatal asphyxia

- Aspiration syndrome (amniotic fluid, meconium)

- Heat loss

- Hypoglycemia

- Polycythemia

- Hypocalcemia

b. Appearance characteristics of the SGA neonate include the following:

**Symmetric IUGR:**
- Head circumference <10th percentile
- Length< 10th percentile
- Proportional body parts
- Weight <10th percentile

**Asymmetric IUGR:**
- Long, thin appearance
- Large appearing head
- Emaciated looking
- Loss of subcutaneous fat
- Loss of muscle mass
- Loose skin folds
- Dry, desquamating skin
- Thin cord
- Decreased chest size
- Decreased abdominal size

c. Consequences for the SGA neonate include a greater risk for mortality or long-term impact of IUGR and/or development of physiologic problems.

d. Assessment for the SGA neonate includes careful assessment of gestational age and assessment for symptoms of the common physiologic problems.

e. Intervention measures include prevention of cold stress and hypoglycemia, parental education, promotion of parent-neonate relationship, and careful monitoring of neonatal response to extrauterine life.

2. **LGA** (Large for Gestational Age) neonates are larger than expected for their gestational age. The term neonate is considered macrosomic if his/her weight is 4000g or more (at or above 90th percentile).

Potential causes of LGA include poorly-controlled maternal diabetes mellitus (White's classification A-C), maternal obesity, genetic predisposition, multiparity, and transposition of the great vessels.

Outcome for the LGA neonate is often a cesarean birth due to CPD or breech position.

a. Common physiologic problems of the LGA neonate include the following:

 – Hypoglycemia

 – Polycythemia

 – Fractured clavicle (due to shoulder dystocia)

 – Brachial plexus palsy (due to shoulder dystocia)

Common physiologic problems of the IDM (Infant of the Diabetic Mother) include the problems of the LGA neonate plus hypocalcemia, hyperbilirubinemia, respiratory distress syndrome, and congenital anomalies.

b. Appearance characteristics of the LGA neonate include the following:

 – Head circumference above the 90th percentile

 – Length above the 90th percentile

 – Weight above the 90th percentile

 – Chubby appearance

c. Consequences for the LGA neonate include birth trauma, CPD, and cesarean birth.

d. Assessment activities for the LGA neonate include gestational age assessment and assessment for common problems of the LGA and IDM neonate. Careful assessment of glucose levels in the IDM neonate during the first 24 hours is essential (because of the intrauterine development of fetal hyperinsulinism).

e. Intervention measures for the LGA neonate include evaluating the neonate's responses and adaptation to extrauterine life, promoting parent-neonate relationship development, and parental education regarding occurrence of any of the common problems and their treatment.

3. **Preterm** neonates are born before completion of 37 weeks gestation. Causes of preterm neonates are not always determined but include the same causes as preterm labor (see Unit 2, Chapter 4: "Selected Intrapartal Complications").

Outcome for preterm neonates is increased mortality and morbidity.

a. Common physiologic problems of the preterm neonate Include the following:

- Patent ductus arteriosus

- Apnea

- Intraventricular hemorrhage

- Retinopathy of prematurity

- Neurologic defects

- Sensorineural hearing loss

- Necrotizing intercolitis

b. Appearance characteristics of the preterm neonate include the following:

- Head appears large in relation to other body parts

- Skin color can be ruddy, cyanotic, or pink

- Skin is translucent with readily visible vessels

- Lack of subcutaneous fat

- Plentiful lanugo

- Nails soft

- Pliable ears

- Small genitalia

- Flaccid tone (frog-like position)

- Weak cry

- Weak, absent, or uncoordinated suck, swallow, and gag reflexes

c. Consequences for the preterm neonate involve the process of adapting to extrauterine life with all immature organ systems.

d. Assessment activities include careful assessment of gestational age, assessment for the common problems of the preterm neonate, and assessment of physiologic instability and stability (preterm neonatal status changes rapidly).

e. Intervention measures include maintaining respiratory function, maintaining cardiovascular function, maintaining a neutral thermal environment and neonatal temperature, maintaining nutrition and fluid/electrolyte balance (including intravenous infusion, gavage feeding), maintaining renal function, maintaining hematologic status, preventing infection, preventing fatigue (especially during feeding, crying), promoting sensory stimulation while avoiding sensory overload, promoting parent-neonate relationship development, educating parents regarding neonate's status and progress, preparing of parents for discharge care (including infant CPR) and follow-up.

4. **Postterm** neonates are born after 42 weeks gestation. The cause of postterm birth is unknown (see Unit 2, Chapter 4: "Selected Intrapartal Complications"). The postterm neonate may be classified as AGA, LGA, or SGA.

Outcome for the postterm neonate includes increased morbidity and mortality due to progressive placental insufficiency.

a. Common physiologic problems of the postterm neonate include the following:

- Birth asphyxia

- Hypoglycemia

- Meconium aspiration syndrome

- Cold stress

- Polycythemia and hyperbilirubinemia

- Seizure activity

b. Appearance characteristics of the postterm neonate include the following:

- Parchment-like, desquamating skin

- No lanugo

- No vernix caseosa

- Long fingernails

- Long, skinny body

- Loose skin

- Lack of subcutaneous fat

- Abundant scalp hair

- Alert facial expression

- Meconium-stained cord and skin

c. Consequences for the postterm neonate include hypoxia and anoxia during labor with an increased risk of fetal demise during labor.

d. Assessment activities for the postterm neonate include assessment for meconium staining of the skin and cord, gestational age assessment, assessment for symptoms of common physiologic problems, and assessment for physiologic stability (especially glucose levels and oxygenation).

e. Intervention measures for the postterm neonate include careful evaluation of adaptation to extrauterine life, prevention of cold stressing, prevention of hypoglycemia, promotion of nutrition, promotion of parent-neonate relationship development, and explanation to parents of appearance of the neonate and any of the common problems the neonate develops.

# PHYSIOLOGICAL PROBLEMS

**Physiological problems** involve neonates with birth asphyxia, respiratory distress, cold stress, hypoglycemia, hyperbilirubinemia, polycythemia, infection, inborn errors of metabolism, and congenital anomalies. Each is summarized as follows.

1. **Birth asphyxia** is failure of the neonate to make the transition to adult-like circulation at birth or interruption of transition to adult-like circulation with resultant decrease in PO2, increase in PCO2, and decrease in pH (acidosis).

The cause can be any of the causes of chronic intrauterine hypoxia or any of the causes of neonatal apnea. Maternal risk factors associated with perinatal asphyxia include PIH, cardiac disease, diabetes mellitus, renal disease, maternal drug use, anemia, and gestational infection (such as toxoplasmosis, cytomegalovirus, or rubella). Other conditions associated with birth asphyxia include prolapsed or compressed cord, impaired fetal circulation, severe respiratory depression due to maternal narcotic administration, placenta previa, abruptio placenta, prematurity, and postmaturity.

Outcome of neonatal asphyxia depends on the early identification of the problem, early initiation of CPR, and the neonate's response to CPR interventions.

a. Symptoms of neonatal asphyxia include the following:

- Cord blood pH of 7.20 or less

- Low Apgar score

- Slow and irregular or absent respiratory efforts

- Cyanosis

- Flaccid muscle tone

- Hypoxemia

     –  Hypercarbia

**b.** Consequences can be negative results of CPR such as irreversible brain changes resulting in damage or death.

**c.** Assessment activities include review of maternal prenatal and labor history for risk factors; cord blood values; Apgar score values; neonatal physiological appearance at birth; and blood gas determination.

**d.** Intervention measures include preparation for immediate neonatal CPR at the moment of birth, preparation of a neutral thermal environment, and preparation of parents for CPR intervention.

2. **Respiratory distress** in the neonate can be classified according to the cause. There are four types: Respiratory Distress Syndrome (RDS) Type I, RDS Type II, Meconium Aspiration Syndrome (MAS), and Persistent Pulmonary Hypertension (PPHN). Each is summarized as follows:

    **a.** RDS Type I (Hyaline Membrane Disease) is idiopathic respiratory distress caused by insufficient surfactant production most often due to immaturity of the lungs in the preterm neonate.

    Outcome for RDS Type I depends on the severity of the disease and the occurrence of other complications and can include an increased risk for mortality and morbidity (bronchopulmonary dysplasia and retinopathy of prematurity).

    **(1)** Symptoms of RDS Type I include as follows:

     –  Rapid (>60 rpm at rest), labored respirations

     –  Cyanosis or pallor

     –  Lower chest and/or xiphoid retractions

     –  Nasal flaring

     –  Grunting

     –  See-saw breathing

     –  Hypotonia

     –  No activity

    **(2)** Consequences of RDS Type I include hypoxemia, respiratory acidosis, and metabolic acidosis.

    **(3)** Assessment activities for RDS Type I include careful assessment for symptoms of RDS Type I, especially increase in cyanosis or pallor, tachypnea, retractions, nasal flaring, grunting respirations, and apnea; and blood gas results.

**(4)** Intervention measures for RDS Type I include maintaining a neutral thermal environment, nutrition, respirations, and cardiac function; prevention of infection; promotion of parent-neonate relationship development; and parental education and emotional support.

**b.** RDS Type II is transient tachypnea of the newborn (TTN) that occurs a short time following birth and is caused by retained lung fluid.

Outcome of RDS Type II is usually improvement by 24-48 hours and completion of the duration of the problem in about 4 days.

**(1)** Symptoms of RDS Type II are very similar to those of RDS Type I except that the neonate is usually a term or near term neonate who experienced intrauterine asphyxia and rarely experiences difficulty with the onset of breathing. Symptoms usually occur during the transition phase of extrauterine adaptation and include the following:

   − Mild cyanosis

   − Nasal flaring

   − Grunting

   − Tachypnea

**(2)** Consequences of RDS Type II usually are minimal.

**(3)** Assessment activities include assessment for increase in the symptoms of RDS Type II, blood gases, and response to treatment.

**(4)** Intervention measures for RDS Type II include parental education and emotional support; promotion of parent-neonate relationship development; and maintaining a neutral thermal environment, nutrition, respiratory function, and cardiac function.

**c.** MAS (Meconium Aspiration Syndrome) is aspiration of meconium stained amniotic fluid. Neonates believed to be at risk for MAS are term SGA or postterm. Release of meconium by the fetus into the amniotic fluid is thought to be caused by intrauterine hypoxia and/or asphyxia. Prevention of MAS can be achieved by use of amnioinfusion to prevent cord compression with resulting hypoxia and/or asphyxia and release of meconium into the amniotic fluid.

Outcome for MAS depends on the ability of the neonate to maintain homeostasis. Inability of the neonate to maintain homeostasis and to remove the meconium from the lungs places the neonate at increased risk for mortality and morbidity.

**(1)** Symptoms of MAS include the following:

- Fetal hypoxia

- Meconium stained amniotic fluid

- Low Apgar scores

- Cyanosis and pallor

- Bradycardia

- Apnea

- Meconium stained skin, cord, nails

**(2)** Consequences of MAS include physical obstruction of the neonatal airways, extreme hypoxia, metabolic acidosis, and respiratory acidosis.

**(3)** Assessment activities for MAS include assessment for symptoms of MAS, blood gas values, and worsening of the neonate's physical status or development of complications of MAS.

**(4)** Intervention measures include parental education and emotional support, promotion of parent-neonate interaction, physiological support (neutral thermal environment, gas exchange, cardiac support, nutrition), and procedures and medications for treatment methods (including extracorporeal membrane oxygenation [ECMO]).

**d.** PPHN is Persistent Pulmonary Hypertension of the Newborn caused by continued pulmonary vascular resistance that results in continued right to left shunting (persistent fetal circulation pattern). It occurs in near-term, term or postterm neonates who have experienced hypoxemia and acidosis insults due to RDS, MAS, Group B streptococcal sepsis, pneumonia, intrapartal asphyxia, or diaphragmatic hernia.

Outcome for PPHN depends on the success of medical intervention to reduce pulmonary vascular resistance.

**(1)** Symptoms of PPHN usually begin by 12-24 hours of age and include the following:

- Tachypnea

- Nasal flaring

- Grunting

- Cyanosis

- Increased anteroposterior chest diameter

- Failure to respond to administration of oxygen

**(2)** Consequences of PPHN include right to left shunting across the ductus arteriosus and/or increased hypoxemia, and further increase in pulmonary vascular resistance.

The neonate is at increased risk for mortality and morbidity (pneumothorax).

**(3)** Assessment for PPHN includes assessment for symptoms of PPHN, rapid change in physiologic status, change in color caused by stimulation or agitation of the neonate, response to treatment procedures and medications, and assessment for symptoms of pneumothorax resulting from aggressive ventilation.

**(4)** Intervention measures for PPHN include maintenance of neutral thermal environment and physiologic functions, planning intervention and assessment activities with minimal disturbance of the neonate, education and emotional support of the parents, and promotion of parent-infant interaction.

3. **Cold stress** is the use of the compensatory mechanisms by the neonate to generate heat in response to excessive heat loss. The cause is excessive heat loss due to evaporation, radiation, conduction, or convection.

Outcome of cold stress is development of respiratory distress and metabolic alterations which can result in death.

   a. Symptoms of cold stress include the following:
   - Increased respiratory rate
   - Decreased skin temperature
   - Peripheral vasoconstriction
   - Acrocyanosis
   - Mottling of the skin
   - Hypoglycemia
   - Metabolic acidosis (late)

   b. Consequences of cold stress include depletion of brown fat and glycogen stores, development of acidosis, decreased surfactant production, and exhaustion.

   c. Assessment activities for cold stress include assessment for symptoms of cold stress and neonatal response to rewarming interventions (continuous assessment of the temperature with a skin probe or axillary temperatures every 15 minutes) during the rewarming process.

    **d.** Intervention measures for cold stress include ideally preventing cold stress through any of the heat loss mechanisms, gradual rewarming to prevent apnea and overheating, maintenance of a neutral thermal environment, and parental education.

**4. Hypoglycemia** is a blood glucose level <40mg/dL. Risk factors for neonatal hypoglycemia include IUGR, postmaturity, IDM, and prematurity.

Outcome for untreated hypoglycemia can be irreversible CNS damage or death.

    **a.** Symptoms of hypoglycemia include the following:

       – Apnea, tachypnea, irregular respirations

       – Cyanosis, pallor

       – Hypotonia, floppy posture

       – Tremors, jitteriness, seizures

       – Lethargy, poor feeding

       – Weak cry, high pitched cry

    **b.** Consequences of hypoglycemia include increased risk for hypothermia and respiratory distress.

    **c.** Assessment activities include assessment of blood glucose levels of at risk neonates, for symptoms of hypoglycemia, and for effectiveness of interventions.

    **d.** Intervention measures include prevention (early feedings of at risk neonates, maintenance of a neutral thermal environment), administration of glucose, maintenance of nutrition, and explanation of the problem and treatment to the parents.

**5. Hyperbilirubinemia** is yellow discoloration of the skin (jaundice) caused by the deposit of unconjugated bilirubin in lipid tissues. There are 2 types of jaundice, physiological jaundice and pathological jaundice.

Physiological jaundice is a bilirubin level of 13 mg/dL or less and is caused by increased RBC lysis due to a normal neonatal biologic response. It appears AFTER the first 24 hours of life and bilirubin levels increase by less than 5 mg/dL per day. See Unit 4, Chapter 1:"Physiologic and Developmental Adaptations" for summarization of bilirubin conjugation and Chapter 3: "Nursing Intervention" for summarization of phototherapy.

Pathological jaundice is an elevated bilirubin level (hyperbilirubinemia) that occurs BEFORE 24 hours of age, exceeds 13 mg/dL, increases more than 5 mg/dL per day, and is most often caused by hemolytic disease of the newborn due to Rh or ABO incompatibility. Other causes are polycythemia, cephalhematoma, and infections.

Outcome for untreated hyperbilirubinemia (pathological jaundice) can be kernicterus (neurologic damage due to deposit of bilirubin in the basal ganglia of the brain).

a. Symptoms of hyperbilirubinemia include the following:

- Jaundice before 24 hours of age

- Bilirubin level >13 mg/dL

- Serum bilirubin level increase of >5 mg/dL/day

- Change in behavior (sleep or appetite)

b. Consequences of hyperbilirubinemia include anemia and increased risk for kernicterus.

c. Assessment activities include review of maternal history for risk factors (Rh negative, blood type), Coomb's test results, neonatal blood type and Rh, bilirubin level, jaundice level (extent of body involved), and effectiveness of treatment interventions.

d. Intervention measures include early feedings to stimulate colonization of intestinal flora and evacuation of meconium, preparation for treatment methods (phototherapy, blood exchange), explanation of treatment method to parents, and promotion of parent-neonate interaction (see Unit 4, Chapter 3: "Nursing Intervention" for phototherapy interventions).

6. **Polycythemia** is increased hematocrit level of 65% or greater most often caused by increased fetal production of RBCs in response to intrauterine hypoxia (caused by any of the causes of placenta insufficiency) or IDM.

Outcome of polycythemia includes hyperviscosity and its consequences (impaired circulation, hyperbilirubinemia, renal vein thrombosis).

a. Symptoms of polycythemia include the following:

- Ruddy appearance

- Hematocrit 65% or greater

- Respiratory distress symptoms

- Hyperbilirubinemia symptoms

- Tachycardia

- Congestive heart failure (CHF) symptoms

- Decreased peripheral pulses

– Oliguria, hematuria, or proteinuria

**b.** Consequences of polycythemia include risk of developing complications due to polycythemia (RDS, CHF, renal vein thrombus, hyperbilirubinemia, seizures).

**c.** Assessment activities for polycythemia include assessment of neonatal admission hematocrit level, symptoms of polycythemia, and treatment response.

**d.** Intervention measures include preparation for treatment procedures (partial blood exchange), education of the parents, maintenance of neonatal physiological functions, and promotion of parent-neonate interactions.

**7. Infection** in the neonate can be caused by organisms acquired from the mother or from health care professionals (primarily due to lack of or poor handwashing techniques). Common organisms and the diseases that they cause in the neonate are listed below:

| ORGANISM | DISEASE |
|---|---|
| Group B Streptococcus | Severe RDS |
| Spirochetes | Congenital Syphilis |
| Gonococci | Ophthalmia Neonatorum |
| Chlamydia Trachomatis | Conjunctivitis and Pneumonia |
| Herpes Type 2 | Neonatal Herpesvirus Infection |
| Candida | Thrush |
| Gram Negative | Sepsis Neonatorum |
| Gram Positive | Sepsis Neonatorum |

Outcome of neonatal infection include increased morbidity and mortality, depending on the organism and disease.

**a.** Symptoms of neonatal infection are specific to the disease.

**b.** Consequences of neonatal infection range all the way to CNS damage and death.

**c.** Assessment activities for neonatal infection include review of maternal history for risk factors; assessment of neonatal skin, oropharynx, and eyes for lesions; observation of neonatal behavioral or appetite changes; temperature instability; apnea; and hyperbilirubinemia.

**d.** Intervention measures include prevention first (handwashing), education of parents, administration of medications and treatment procedures, promotion of neonatal physiological functions, emotional support of parents, and promotion of parent-neonate interaction.

8. **Inborn errors of metabolism** are hereditary disorders that Cause alteration in metabolism due to lack of specific enzymes. The most common inborn error of metabolism is phenylketonuria (PKU) and others include maple syrup urine disease, galacto-semia, and homocystinuria.

   Outcome of inborn errors of metabolism includes accumulation of toxic metabolites in the neonate with varying consequences.

   a. Symptoms of inborn errors of metabolism are specific to the type of inborn error of metabolism. The neonates appear normal at birth and present with symptoms as the metabolites accumulate in the body. Several of the disorders have CNS symptoms.

   b. Consequences for inborn errors of metabolism vary according to the specific disorder. PKU, the most common disorder, has a consequence of mental retardation if treatment is not insti-tuted. Mothers who as infants/children were successfully treated for PKU (dietary restriction of phenylaline) must resume the dietary restriction before conception and continue the restriction during pregnancy to prevent fetal damage.

   c. Assessment activities for inborn errors of metabolism include completion of the initial newborn screen for several of the disorders (PKU, maple syrup urine disease, homocystinuria, galactosemia) plus sickle cell anemia and congenital hypo-thyroidism before the neonate is dismissed from the hospital.

   d. Intervention measures for inborn errors of metabolism include planning for follow-up assessment, education of parents for dietary management, and referral for support groups.

9. **Congenital anomalies** that are obvious at birth include cleft lip and/or palate, choanal atresia, hydrocephalus, omphalocele, tracheoesophageal fistula, and myelomeningocele.

   Outcome for congenital anomalies depend on the type and the response to surgical correction.

   a. Signs and symptoms are specific to the anomaly.

   b. Consequences of congenital anomalies depend on neonatal response to medical intervention.

   c. Assessment for congenital anomalies include a thorough physical assessment of the neonate, a review of maternal history, and assessment of neonatal response to adaptation to extrauterine life.

   d. Intervention measures for congenital anomalies include preparation for treatment procedures, administration of medi-cations and procedures, preparation of the parents for the anomaly and treatment outcome, emotional support of the parents, promotion of parent-neonate relationship development, and referral to support groups if applicable.

# ACQUIRED PROBLEMS

**Acquired problems** involve neonates with birth trauma, neonates of substance abuse mothers, and neonates at risk for parent-infant relationship problems. Each problem is summarized as follows:

1. **Birth trauma problems** that occur most often are caput succedaneum, cephalhematoma, fractured clavicle, and brachial palsy. See Unit 4, Chapter 1: "Physiological and Developmental Adaptations" for summarization of caput succedaneum and cephalhematoma.

    a. Brachial palsy is injury to the brachial plexus caused by a difficult birth (shoulder dystocia).

    b. Fractured clavicle is a fracture that occurs most often in the middle of the bone and is caused by shoulder dystocia.

    Outcome for brachial palsy and fractured clavicle is usually return of function with healing. However, if the brachial plexus nerve has been lacerated, return of function may not occur.

    c. Symptoms of brachial palsy include the following:
    – Flaccid arm
    – Extension at the elbow
    – Inward rotation of the hand
    – Absence of response to the Moro reflex in the affected arm
    – Intact palmar grasp reflex

    Symptoms of fractured clavicle include the following:
    – Limited motion of the affected arm
    – Bone crepitus
    – Absence of response to the Moro reflex in the affected arm

    d. Assessment activities for brachial plexus and fractured clavicle include review of birth history and assessment for symptoms.

    e. Intervention measures for brachial plexus and fractured clavicle include immobilization of the affected arm, careful handling of the neonate, explanation of the care and expected outcome to the parents, emotional support of the parents in learning to provide neonatal care, and promotion of parent-neonate relationship development.

2 **Substance abuse problems** occur in neonates of mothers with alcohol, illegal drug, and tobacco dependency.

Outcome for tobacco dependency includes decreased birth weight and increased risk for preterm birth.

Outcome for alcohol and illegal drug dependency includes the teratogenic effect on the fetus and often the effect of placental insufficiency.

   a. Symptoms of tobacco dependency include symptoms of symmetric IUGR.

   Symptoms of alcohol drug dependency (Fetal Alcohol Syndrome [FAS]) include the following:

   – IUGR symptoms

   – Microcephaly

   – Irritability/Hyperactivity

   – Congenital anomalies

   – Characteristic facial features

   – Withdrawal symptoms

   Symptoms of illegal drug dependency includes the following:

   – IUGR symptoms

   – Hyperirritability

   – Tremor, seizures

   – Poor feeding

   – Rapid shift from irritability to lethargy

   – Temperature elevation

   – Respiratory distress

   – Hyperreflexia

   – Vomiting, drooling

   – Sensitive gag reflex

   – Diarrhea, abdominal cramps

   – Stuffy nose, sneezing, yawning

   – Flushing, sweating

   – Circumoral pallor

   – Congenital anomalies

b. Consequences of tobacco abuse include residual growth deficits, intellectual and emotional developmental deficits, deficits in behavior, and increased risk for prematurity. In addition, neonates and children exposed to secondhand smoke have more URI, bronchitis, and asthma.

Consequences of FAS include CNS effects (mental retardation, hyperactivity), growth deficiency, facial abnormalities, congenital anomalies, and alcohol withdrawal.

Consequences of illegal drug dependency include neonatal complications (respiratory distress, hyperbilirubinemia), growth deficiencies, poor state organization (rapid shift between states), congenital anomalies, drug withdrawal, greater risk of Sudden Infant Death Syndrome, greater risk of GI and respiratory illnesses, and behavioral problems.

c. Assessment includes review of maternal health history and birthing history, careful physical behavioral assessment, and assessment for symptoms of withdrawal.

d. Intervention measures for substance abuse includes treatment for neonatal withdrawal, administration of medications, maintenance of physiological functions and stability, promotion of parent-neonate relationship development, and planning for follow-up evaluation.

3. **Parent-infant relationship problems** involve alterations in parenting of the infant. The causes are numerous. Risk factors include abnormal pregnancy, abnormal birthing process, mother-neonate/infant separation, and maternal or neonatal/infant illness.

Outcome of alteration in parent-infant relationship development can be neglect and/or abuse.

a. Symptoms of parent-infant relationship problems include the following:

— Lack of interest in the pregnancy

— Lack of interest in fetal well-being

— Lack of interest in seeing or touching the neonate

— Negative comments about the neonatal sex or characteristics

— Refusal to care for the neonate

b. Consequences of parent-neonate relationship problems include failure-to-thrive complications.

c. Assessment activities for parent-neonate relationship problems include careful review of maternal prenatal and birthing process attitude and verbalizations, assessment of cultural practices for childbearing, assessment of family dynamics, assessment of family financial status and support system, and assessment of parental expectations regarding parenting this specific neonate.

d. Intervention measures for parent-neonate relationship problems include supporting maternal grieving for differences between her "fantasy" neonate and her real neonate, emotional support, role modeling caretaking behavior, identifying positive neonatal characteristics, and referral to a support group or person.

# APPENDIX A
# SUMMARY OF CONTRACEPTIVE METHODS

*Contraception is the prevention, planning, and/or spacing of pregnancies based on the couple's choice to either not have children or to select the number of children desired and the timing for the birth of each child. A variety of methods are available to couples. In order to make an informed choice of method, the couple needs to know the mode of action, effectiveness, advantages, disadvantages, side effects, indications, contraindications, and requirements for use of the methods. Contraceptive methods can be classified as oral contraceptives, spermicides, barrier methods, long-acting methods, voluntary sterilization, and fertility awareness methods. Basic information for commonly used contraceptive methods is summarized below.*

## Oral Contraception

**Mode of Action** of oral contraception is primarily inhibition of ovulation with combination (estrogen and progestin) pills. Other changes caused by oral contraceptive pills include alteration of the cervical mucus, endometrial lining, and tubal transport.

**Effectiveness** as measured by the expected first-year reported failure rate is 0.1% (Hatcher et al., 1994).

**Advantages** of oral contraception include the following:

- Safety (for most women)

- Timing of next menses is known

- Less menstrual flow

- Relief of menstrual cycle problems (cramps, pain)

- Spontaneity of intercourse (method not associated with intercourse)

- Protection against acute pelvic inflammatory disease

- Protection against ovarian and endometrial cancer

- Prevention of ectopic pregnancy

- Improvement of acne

- Suppression of functional ovarian cysts

- Prevention of benign breast cysts and fibroadenomas
- Excellent reversibility

**Disadvantages** of oral contraception include the following:
− Pill must be taken daily at the same time (motivation)

− No protection against STDs

− No protection against Human Immunodeficiency Virus (HIV)

− Expense (for some women)

− Side effects

− Decreased effectiveness with other medications (antibiotics, anti-convulsants)

**Side effects** associated with oral contraception include the following:
− Spotting or breakthrough bleeding

− Breast fullness/tenderness (in some women)

− Nausea (with first packet or first few pills of each pack)

− Mood changes (in some women)

− Chloasma (in some women)

− Headaches (in some women)

− Circulatory complications (rare)

− Increased risk of liver tumors (rare)

**Indications** for oral contraception include the following:
* Sexually-active young women and adolescents

* Nulliparous women

* Spacing of pregnancies

* Nonlactating postpartal women

* Acne

* Heavy or painful menses

* Recurrent ovarian cysts

* Family history of ovarian cancer

**Contraindications** for oral contraception include the following:
* Thromboembolic disease

* Cerebrovascular accident

* Coronary artery disease

* Breast cancer

* Estrogen-dependent neoplasia

* Pregnancy

* Liver tumor

* Impaired liver function

* Previous cholestasis during pregnancy

**Requirements for use** include the ability to take the pill daily and to follow instructions for missing a pill.

# Spermicides

Spermicide methods include foams, creams, gels, tablets (vaginal), film, and suppositories.

**Mode of Action** for spermicides is a chemical (usually Nonoxynol-9) that kills the sperm.

**Effectiveness** of spermicides as measured by the first-year failure rate among perfect users is a failure rate of 6% and a typical failure rate of 21% (Hatcher et al., 1994). Spermicides are most effective when used in combination with a barrier method.

**Advantages** of spermicide include the following:

* Can be purchased over the counter

* Simple backup method for other contraceptive methods

* Provide lubrication

* Simple temporary method

* Protection against some sexually transmitted diseases (especially gonorrhea)

**Disadvantages** for spermicides include the following:

– Messy

– Typical failure rate of 21%

– Use is associated with intercourse

**Side Effects** for spermicides include temporary skin irritation in some users.

**Indications** for spermicides include temporary need, backup method need, and need for a method without a prescription.

**Contraindications** for spermicides include allergy to ingredients, inability to correctly use the spermicide, and vaginal abnormality that prevents placement and retention of spermicide in the vagina so that it covers the cervix.

Requirements for use of spermicides include use of the method for each episode of sexual intercourse and leaving spermicide in the vagina for 6-8 hours after intercourse (douching is not necessary).

## Barrier Methods

Barrier methods include condoms, the diaphragm, the sponge, and the cervical cap.

**Mode of Action** of barrier methods includes a mechanical barrier to prevent transportation of the sperm to the ovum.

**Effectiveness** of barrier methods as measured by typical failure rates for first-year use is a failure rate of 5%-26% (Hatcher et al., 1994). Effectiveness is improved when barrier methods are combined with spermicides.

**Advantages** of barrier methods include the following:

- Inexpensive

- Safe

- No prescription required (accessible)

- Health provider intervention not required (except for diaphragm and cap)

- Provide some protection against STDs

- Prevents messiness of seminal discharge in the vagina

**Disadvantages** of barrier methods include the following:
- Defective device

- Use is associated with sexual intercourse

- Device must be used with each episode of intercourse

**Side effects** of barrier methods include the following:
* Skin irritation (in some users with some methods)

* Difficulty removing the sponge

* Vaginal dryness with the sponge

* Possible increase in yeast infections with the sponge

* Increased risk of urinary tract infection with the diaphragm

* Possible pap smear abnormalities with the cervical cap

**Indications** for use of barrier methods include need for a temporary method, a backup method, and/or an easily accessible method.

**Contraindications** for use of barrier methods include the following:

* Allergy to rubber, latex, polyurethane, or chemicals in the sponge

* Inability to learn correct insertion/application technique

* History of toxic shock syndrome

* Repeated urinary tract infections

**Requirements for use** of barrier methods include motivation to use the method with each act of intercourse and ability to correctly insert or apply and remove the device. The diaphragm must be left in place at least 6 hours (until the spermicide kills the sperm) after intercourse, the condom must be held in place over the penis when the penis is withdrawn, and additional applications of spermicide must be used if intercourse is repeated before the end of 6-8 hours when the diaphragm is used.

# LONG-ACTING METHODS

Long-acting methods include progestin-only implants (norplant) or injections and intrauterine devices (IUDs). Each method is summarized below.

## Progestin-only methods

**Mode of Action** for progestin-only methods is primarily inhibition of ovulation. Other changes include thickening of cervical mucus, atrophic endometrium, and luteolysis.

**Effectiveness** of progestin-only methods as measured by perfect use is 0.09% to 1.5% (Hatcher et al., 1994).

**Advantages** of progestin-only, long-acting methods include the following:

• Highly effective

• Method is not associated with intercourse

• Method is long-acting (5 years for implant, 3 months for injection)

• Easily reversible (implant)

• No estrogen-related side effects

• Scanty or no menses (in some women)

• Decreased menses cramping and pain (in some women)

• Does not suppress lactation

**Disadvantages** of progestin-only long-acting methods include the following:

− Menstrual cycle irregularities (amenorrhea)

— Reversibility may be delayed (injection)

— Implant may be slightly visible

— Initial expense for implant is high

— Implant requires minor surgery for insertion and removal

— Injections required for injectable progestin

**Side effects** of the progestin-only long-acting methods include the following:

* Menstrual irregularities

**Indications** for long-term, progestin-only contraception include the following:

* Continuous contraception

* Long-term spacing of births

* Desire no more births

* Do not desire sterilization

* Experienced side effects with other contraception methods

* Lactation

**Contraindications** for long-term progestin-only contraception include the following:

* Acute liver disease

* Jaundice

* Unexplained, undiagnosed vaginal bleeding

* Thrombophlebitis or pulmonary embolism

* Cardiac disease or cerebrovascular disease

**Requirements for use** include returning for removal of the implant in five years and returning for progestin injection every three months.


## IUDs

**Mode of Action** for the IUD is not completely understood but may be due to the effect on the sperm, ova, fertilization, implantation, endometrium and/or fallopian tube.

**Effectiveness** of the IUD as measured by the first-year failure rate is 0.1% to 1.5% (Hatcher et al., 1994).

**Advantages** of the IUD method include the following:
- Long-acting contraception

- Method not associated with intercourse

**Disadvantages** of the IUD include the following:
- Must be inserted and removed by a health provider

- Increased menstrual bleeding (in some women)

- Dysmenorrhea (in some women)

**Side Effects** of the IUD include the following:
* Expulsion (in some women during the first year)

* Uterine/cervical perforation or embedding (rare)

* Increased risk for pelvic inflammatory disease (PID) (in the first few weeks following insertion in some women)

**Indications** for IUDs include the following:
* Multiparous women

* Monogamous relationships

**Contraindications** for the IUD include the following absolute, relative, and possible relative contraindications:
**Absolute** (method is not prescribed):
* PID

* Pregnancy

**Relative** (not prescribed unless other methods are even less desirable):
* Postpartum or postabortion infection

* Purulent cervicitis

* Recurrent gonorrhea

* STD risk factors (multiple partners or partner with multiple sex partners)

* Undiagnosed irregular bleeding

* Ectopic pregnancy history

* Impaired coagulation

**Other relative** (prescribed with careful monitoring):
* Valvular heart disease

* Uterine anomalies

* Menstrual disorder

* Anemia

**Requirements for use** include checking for the presence of the strings (weekly the first month and after each menses), compliance with recommended follow-up check-ups, and compliance with recommended removal.

## Sterilization

Voluntary sterilization methods include vasectomy (men) and tubal ligation or blockage (women).

**Mode of Action** is prevention of ova transport through the fallopian tube (tubal ligation) and prevention of sperm transport through the vas deferens (vasectomy).

**Effectiveness** as measured by failure rates include a failure rate of less than 1% (Hatcher et al., 1994).

**Advantages** of sterilization include the following:

• Permanent

• Highly effective

• Safe

• Economical

**Disadvantages** of sterilization include the following:

− Irreversible

− Minor surgical procedure

**Side effects** of sterilization include complications of the surgical procedure (infection, bleeding, anesthesia).

**Indications** for sterilization include the following:

\* Personal preference

\* Multiparity

\* Medical disorders

\* Hereditary disease

**Contraindications** for sterilization include the following:

\* Youth (<21 years of age if federal funds are used)

\* Mental incompetence

**Requirements for use** includes informed consent before deciding to proceed with the sterilization.

# Fertility Awareness Methods

Fertility awareness methods include calendar, basal body temperature, and cervical mucus charting, or a combination of one or more of the methods.

**Mode of Action** for the fertility awareness methods is abstinence from sexual intercourse during the fertile period of the menstrual cycle.

**Effectiveness** for the fertility awareness methods as measured by the typical user during the first-year of use is a failure rate of approximately 20% (Hatcher et al., 1994).

**Advantages** of the fertility awareness methods include the following:

• Safety

• No cost

• No religious objections

• Promote learning about body functions

• Useful to plan a pregnancy (time intercourse during fertile period)

**Disadvantages** of fertility awareness methods include the following:

– Extensive abstinence for irregular menstrual cycles

– Extensive counseling to learn to use the methods correctly

**Side effects** for the fertility awareness methods include frustration during periods of abstinence.

**Indications** for use of fertility awareness methods include personal or religious desire to use a "natural" method and willingness to accept an unplanned pregnancy.

**Contraindications** for use of fertility awareness methods include the following:

* Irregular menstrual cycles

* Anovulatory menstrual cycles

* Irregular temperature chart results

* Unwillingness to use abstinence during the fertile period

* Inability to keep accurate charts

**Requirements for use** of the fertility awareness methods include motivation to correctly use the method and learning how to correctly use the method.

# Reference

Hatcher, R.A., Trussell, J., Stewart, F., Stewart, G.K., Kowal, D., Guest, F., and Cates, W., and Policar, M.S. (1994). *Contraceptive Technology (1994).* New York: Irvington Publishers, Inc.

# APPENDIX B
# ADOLESCENT PREGNANCY AND PARENTING

**Adolescence** is the transition period between childhood and adulthood. During the transition, the adolescent completes several milestones, such as physical maturity (beginning with the onset of puberty), cognitive development, independence from parents, and a personal identity. Puberty onset currently ranges from 9-14 years of age and the adolescent becomes aware of body changes plus increasing sexual hormone levels. Thus, the adolescent is at risk for engaging in risky behaviors as he/she responds to physical, hormonal, and developmental changes. High risk behaviors include unprotected sexual intercourse and multiple sex partners over time.

a. **Consequences** of selected risky behaviors include the following:

- STDs

  - HIV infection

  - premature death related to AIDS

  - increased risk of developing pelvic inflammatory disease which can impair future fertility capability (for females only)

- Adolescent Pregnancy

  - complications of pregnancy and low birth weight infant

  - interrupted/terminated educational preparation
  - repeated adolescent pregnancies

  - single parenthood

b. **Assessment** during adolescent pregnancy includes the following:

- the standard pregnancy assessments (see Prenatal Period Maternal and Fetal Assessment)

- risk factors for complications of pregnancy (PIH, preterm labor, STDs, spontaneous abortion, intrauterine growth retardation)

- nutritional status (anemia, inadequate weight gain)

- completion of the developmental tasks of pregnancy (acceptance of the pregnancy, fetus/neonate, and parenting role)

- support network (partner, family, social groups)

- psycho-social status

- sexual abuse (may lead to alcohol/substance abuses, late prenatal care enrollment, skipping prenatal appointments, physical abuse during pregnancy)

- sexuality and reproductive knowledge base

c. **Interventions** during adolescent pregnancy implemented in a nonjudgmental, caring approach include the following:

- early, regular, continuing prenatal care (to identify causes of poor pregnancy outcomes; initiate preventive/treatment measures to eliminate/reduce consequences)

- referral to social support services (as needed to prevent/reduce negative effects of a less than optimal socioeconomic environment and/or support network)

- adolescent-oriented prenatal education (pregnancy, labor, postpartum, newborn, early parenting, early grandparenting)

- nutrition counseling (to meet adolescent and pregnancy growth needs, necessity of achieving recommended weight gain utilizing high nutrient foods)

**Adolescent Parenthood** may be a reality shock for the adolescent (she may have perceived that her problem was the pregnancy and that as soon as the pregnancy was over, her problem would "go away"), can result in developmental conflicts (meeting responsibilities of parenthood versus experiencing "fun" activities with peers), and frequently results in frustration (especially related to unrealistic age expectations of the infant/child, demands and needs of the infant/child, and self-view of parenting role expectations versus reality). Thus, ongoing assessment and intervention is required following birth of the neonate.

a. **Assessments** for adolescent parenting include the following:

- maternal role (definition, expectations, attitude)
- problem-solving capabilities
- decision-making process
- self-concept
- mother-infant/child interaction (verbal and nonverbal)
- mother-infant/child relationship development
- care-giver task capability (bathing, feeding, diapering/dressing, wellness care, illness care)
- stress level
- coping strategies
- financial support
- educational plans/expectations
- support network

b. **Interventions** for adolescent parenting include the following:
- anticipatory guidance
- development of a cooperative, trusting client-nurse relationship

- developmentally focused education (mother and infant/child, maternal wellness/illness assessment skills, physical and cognitive abilities)

- role modeling (self-care and infant/child care and interaction [verbal and nonverbal])

- nutrition teaching (mother and infant/child)

- referrals (financial, social, developmental services)

- case management

# APPENDIX C
# HOME CARE

**Home Care Nursing Practice** is defined as "... a unique combination of community health and acute care nursing provided in the client's home" (Lowdermilk, et al, 1997, p. 84). The practice may be general (infants to elderly) or specialized (oncologic, pediatric, perinatal, etc.). The employer may be a hospital, hospital system, independent agency, or third party payer.

The American Nurses Association has developed Standards of Home Health Care. The Association of Women's Health, Obstetric and Neonatal Nurses has developed a description of nursing practice for preconception, antepartum, and postpartum home care nursing. In addition, HCFA has further defined perinatal home care nursing practice.

a. **Required nursing knowledge base and skills** for home care include the following:

- case management

- client education

- conditions and characteristics with risk potential for pregnancy complications

- coordination of care

- consultation

- diagnostic studies

- diagnostic and therapeutic technologies and procedures

- decision-making

- employee safety

- evaluation of health status (maternal and fetal)

- general health profile

- health care and other resources availability to client

- health care equipment
- health care supervision
- health education
- home and community assessment
- infection control
- laboratory tests (especially specimen collection)
- management of emergencies
- maternal postpartal adaptation
- medications commonly used in pregnancy (including high risk pregnancy)
- neonatal assessment and care
- pathophysiology of common complications
- physical assessment
- physiologic aspects of high risk pregnancy
- postpartal family adaptation
- professional considerations
- psychosocial adaptation to pregnancy (including at risk pregnancy)
- psychosocial aspects of high risk pregnancy
- regulatory bodies and mandates for practice
- reproductive anatomy and physiology

b. **Strategies** for home care case management include critical paths/pathways, telephone advice lines, electronic data transmission, and home visits.

c. **Client type** for home care management is based on medical diagnosis severity, third party provider criteria, and availability of home care services and may include the following expectant mothers with the following perinatal diagnoses:

- bleeding
- cardiac problems

- diabetes mellitus

- decreased fetal movement

- early post-delivery discharge (mother and neo-nate)

- hydramnios

- hyeremesis gravidarum

- multiple sclerosis

- neonatal jaundice

- pregnancy induced hypertension

- preterm labor

- preterm infant

- small for gestational age infant

d. **Nursing activities** specific to the medical and nursing diagnoses include the following:

- assessments (client, home, safety, environment, community)

- development of a Plan of Care

- formulation of expected client-centered out-comes

- self-care and neonate/infant care education

- evaluation and documentation of care and out-comes

(Please review the selected prenatal, intrapartal, postpartal, and neonatal complications for symptoms, consequences, and interventions.)

# Appendix D
# REFERENCES

Dahlberg, N., Escher-Davis, L., Eaton, D. G., and Stringer, M. (1994). *Didactic Content and Clinical Skills Verification for Professional Nurse Providers of Perinatal Home Care.* Washington, DC: AWHONN.

Hatcher, R.A., Trussell, J., Stewart, F., Stewart, G.K., Kowal, D., Guest, F., Cates, W., and Policar, M.S. (1994). *Contraceptive technology (1994).* New York: Irvington Publishers, Inc.

Lowdermilk, D. L., Perry, S E., and Bobak, I. M. (1997). *Maternity and Women's Health Care.* Sixth Edition. St. Louis: Mosby.

May, K.A. and Mahlmeister, L.R. (1990). *Comprehensive maternity nursing: nursing process and the childbearing family.* Second Edition. New York: J.B. Lippincott Company.

Olds, S.B., London, M.L., and Ladewig, P.W. (1996).*Maternal-new born nursing: a family approach.* Fifth Edition. Menlo Park: Addison-Wesley.

Pillitteri, A. (1992). *Maternal and child health nursing: care of the childbearing and childrearing family.* New York: J.B. Lippincott Company.

Tucker, S.M. (1996). *Pocket guide to fetal monitoring.* Third Edition. St. Louis: Mosby.

# Index

## A

Abdomen, 187
Abortion, 61, 21
amenorrhea, 9
Amniocentesis, 49
amnion, 7
amniotic fluid, 7, 95, 122, 129
Anemia, 61
        Physiologic Anemia of Infancy, 176
        Physiologic of Pregnancy, 12
Anesthesia, 103
antepartum, 21
Anus, 188
Anxiety, 103, 132
Apgar scores, 98, 99, 185, 205, 208
Apgar scoring system, 98
Appetite changes, 14
areolae, 140
Assessment
        Fetal, 30
        Neonate, 99
        Well-being, 29

## B

Back, 188
Backache, 17, 52
Backpain, 64
Ballard Scale, 189
Ballottement, 10
Bilirubin, 178
Bilirubin conjugation, 178
biophysical profile, 31
Birthmarks, 180
bladder, 15
Blood, 139
Blood incompatibility, 69
Blood pressure, 13, 139
blood volume, 12
Body Mass Index, 57
Boggy fundus, 163
bonding, 149
Bony pelvis, 83
Brachial palsy, 214

Bradycardia, 96
Breast, 51, 191
Breast engorgement, 151
Breasts, 12, 138, 147
        self-exam, 58
breech, 110
Breech presentation, 84, 111
Brow presentation, 112
brown fat, 176

# C

Calcium, 16
Carbohydrates, 16
Cardiac disease, 60, 131, 171
Cardiac output, 13, 139
Cardiovascular system adaptations, 175
Carpal tunnel syndrome, 52
Cervix, 12, 95, 137
Cesarean birth, 133
Chadwick's sign, 9, 12
Chest, 187
chloasma, 9, 140
chorion, 7
Circumcision, 198
clotting factors, 13
Coagulation Abnormality, 161
        Disseminated Intravascular Coagulopathy, 161
Cold stress, 177, 196, 209
Colostrum, 138
complications, 105
conception, 3, 6
Conduction, 176
Constipation, 14, 52
Contraction stress test, 46
Contractions, 18, 42, 80, 82, 93, 9, 119
        Braxton-Hicks, 10
Convection, 176
Coomb's Indirect, 70
Corpus luteum, 3, 4, 5, 7, 12, 18
Culture, 19
cystitis, 164
Cystocele, 56

# D

Deceleration, 42

Descent, 88
Developmental Assessment, 148
Diabetes Mellitus, 61, 131, 171
dilatation, 80, 81, 82, 95, 97
Disseminated Intravascular Coagulopathy (DIC), 73, 76
dystocia, 119
Dysuria, 64

**E**

Ear, 191, 192
Early Decelerations, 42
Eclampsia, 76
Edema, 54, 75, 92
Effacement, 81, 95, 97
Electronic Fetal Monitoring (EFM), 32
Electronic monitoring, 93
Elimination, 153
embryo, 7
endometritis, 165
Endometritis, 164
Engagement, 88
Episiotomy, 154
Episiotomy site, 147
Erythema toxicum, 180
Erythroblastosis fetalis, 70
Erythromycin ophthalmic ointment, 195
Estimated Date of Delivery (EDD), 26
Estrogen, 3, 4, 7, 12, 13, 16, 18, 70, 80, 86
Estrogen stimulation theory, 80
Evaporation, 176
Exercise, 56
Expulsion, 89
Extension, 88
Extracorporeal membrane oxygenation (ECMO), 208
Extremities, 188

**F**

face presentation, 112
Faintness, 54
Fallopian tubes, 6
Fatigue, 52
Fertilization, 6
fetal by-passes, 175
Fetal Alcohol Syndrome (FAS), 215
Fetal Assessment, 30

fetal attitude, 84
Fetal baseline, 32
Fetal distress, 115
Fetal Heart rate, 112
fetal heartbeat, 10
fetal lie, 84
Fetal movement, 30
fetal position, 84, 88
        persistent occiput posterior, 113
        persistent occiput posterior , 114
Fetal position, 98
Fetal presentation, 29, 84, 98, 119
Fetal presenting part, 88, 96
fetus, 7
First trimester, 51
Flatulence, 53
flexion, 88
Fluid and Electrolytes, 15
Follicle Stimulating Hormone (FSH), 3, 4
Fundal Height, 92

## G

Gastrin, 14
Gastrointestinal system adaptations, 177
Genitalia, 188
Genitals, 192
Germ layers, 7
Gestation, 21
Gestational Age, 189, 191, 200
        Large for, 201
        Small for, 200
Gestational diabetes, 61, 69, 70, 71
Gonadotropin-releasing hormone (GnRH), 3
Goodell's sign, 10
graafian follicle, 3
Graafian follicle, 4
Gravida, 21
gravity, 141

## H

Head, 186
health history, 22, 23, 24
Heart Sounds, 92
Heartburn, 14, 53
Hegar's sign, 10

HELLP syndrome, 76
hematoma, 159
hematopoietic system, 176
Hemorrhage, 71, 110, 159, 162
Hemorrhoids, 14, 140
Hormones, 17
Human chorionic gonadotropin, 9
Human chorionic gonadotropin (HCG), 7, 18
Human Placental Lactogen (HCL), 7
human placental lactogen (HPL), 18
Hunger, 139
Hyaline Membrane Disease, 206
Hydatidiform mole, 72, 74, 75
hydramnios, 121, 129
Hydrocephaly, 115
Hyperbilirubinemia, 210
Hyperemesis gravidarum, 69, 74
Hyperglycemia, 62
Hyperplasia, 11
Hypertension, 75
        Persistent Pulmonary of the Newborn (PPHN), 208
Hyperthermia, 177
Hyperventilation, 13, 86
Hypoglycemia, 62, 210
Hypotension, 13, 54

# I

Immunity
        Active-acquired, 179
        Passive-acquired, 179
Immunizations, 59
Immunologic system adaptations, 179
infection, 212
Infections, 64, 163
Insomnia, 54
Insulin, 18
Integumentary system adaptations, 179
Intrapartum, 21
Intrauterine growth retardation, 191, 200
iron, 16
Iron storage, 178
ischial spines, 88

# J

Jaundice
  Physiologic, 198

# K

Kegel exercises, 56
kernicterus, 178

# L

Labor, 88, 93, 97, 134
  Augmentation of, 134
  False Signs, 81
  induction of, 134
  postterm, 125
  precipitous, 123
  Premonitory signs of , 81
  preterm, 124,
  prolonged, 122
  stages of, 89, 90
  True signs, 82
Labor patterns
  Hypertonic dysfunctional, 119
  Hypotonic dysfunctional, 121
Laboratory Assessment, 25
Laboratory tests, 92
Lactation, 12
Lanugo, 9, 191, 204
Late Decelerations, 42
Leg cramps, 54
Leopold's maneuvers, 95, 111, 112, 113, 115
letting-go phase, 142
Leukorrhea, 52
Lightening, 81
linea nigra, 9, 140
Linea nigra, 16
lochia, 137, 147, 165
Long-term variability, 38
Lung Sounds, 92
Luteinizing Hormone, 3

# M

Macrosomia, 114, 121
Magnetic Resonance Imaging, 31
Mastitis, 166
Maternal serum alpha-fetoprotein (MSAFP), 50

Maturity Rating, 192
McDonald's sign, 10
Meconium, 177, 204
membranes, 95, 97
Menstrual Cycle, 3, 5
Midpelvic contracture, 106
Milia, 180
Mittelschmerz, 4
Molding, 84
Mood Swings, 20, 52
Multigravida, 21
Multipara, 22
Muscle cramps, 17

## N

Nägele's Rule, 26
Nausea, 14, 51, 64
Neck, 187
Neonatal period, 21, 173
Neonate, 21
Neonates
        postterm, 204
        preterm, 202
Neurologic System Adaptations, 180
Nipple-stimulation stress testing, 46
nitrogen, 16
nocturia, 9
Nulligravida, 22
Nullipara, 22
Nutrition, 57, 153
        Neonatal, 196

## O

oligohydramnios, 130
Ophthalmia Neonatorum, 195
organogenesis, 6, 9
Outlet pelvic contracture, 106
Ovarian cycle, 4
Ovaries, 12, 138
Ovulation, 3, 4, 12
Oxytocin, 18, 80, 86
oxytocin administration, 134
Oxytocin Challenge Test, 49
Oxytocin theory, 80

# P

Para, 22
patent ductus arteriosus, 203
Pathological Retraction ring, 107, 108
Pelvic inlet contracture, 105
pelvis, 105
Percutaneous umbilical blood sampling, 49
Perineum, 138
Peristalsis, 140
Phenylketonuria (PKU), 213
Physical Assessment, 25, 97
Pica, 57
Pigmentation, 140
        Chloasma, 16
PIH/HELLP, 161
PIH/HELLP syndrome, 131
Pituitary changes, 18
Placenta, 7, 8, 12, 14, 85, 126
        abruptio placentae, 72, 76, 126
        placental insufficiency, 126
        placenta previa, 71, 73, 126
        Retained Placental Fragments, 160
Plantar creases, 191
Polycythemia, 211
Popliteal Angle, 190
Positive Symptoms, 10
postpartal period, 135
Postpartum, 22, 169
Postpartum "blues", 168, 170
postpartum hemorrhage, 162
Posture, 189
Preeclampsia, 75
Pregnancy-Induced Hypertension, 69, 75
Prenatal period, 1, 22
Primigravida, 22
Primipara, 22
Progesterone, 4, 6, 7, 12, 14, 15, 18, 70, 86
Progesterone Withdrawal Theory, 80
Prostaglandin, 4, 19
puerperal complications, 157, 162
puerperium, 135, 148
Pulse, 139
Pyelonephritis, 164

# Q

Quickening,  9, 29

# R

Radiation,  176
rectum,  147
Reflexes,  177
    Arm Recoil,  190
    Arm recoil,  181
    Babinski,  181
    Crossed extension,  181
    Head lag,  181
    Landau,  181
    Moro,  180, 185
    Palmar grasp,  214
    Plantar grasp,  180
    Rooting,  180
    Sucking,  180
    Tonic neck,  180
Relaxin,  18, 19, 83
Renal function,  15
Renal system functions,  179
Reproductive system adaptations,  181
Restitution,  89
Rh factor,  70
Risk Factors,  23
Round ligament pain,  53
Rupture of Membranes,  77, 81,  92, 97, 106

# S

Scarf sign,  190
Second Trimester,  52
Second trimester discomforts,  52
Sexual Relations,  57
Sexually transmitted diseases,  64, 65
Shortness of breath,  55
Short-term variability,  38
Skin,  186, 190, 191
sleep phase,
Spinnbarkeit,  4, 6
Square window,  189
station,  95
Stillbirth,  22
Stretch Theory,  80
striae,  9, 12, 15

striae gravidarum, 140
Substance abuse, 56, 215
Sudden Infant Death Syndrome, 216
Supine hypotension, 13, 53, 102
Surfactant, 174
Symptoms of Pregnancy
    Positive, 10
    Presumptive, 9
    Probable, 9

# T

Tachycardia, 96
taking-hold phase, 142, 149
taking-in phase, 142, 149
Teratogens, 9
thermal neutral zone, 177
Third trimester , 54
Thirst, 139
Thrombophlebitis, 166, 167
thyroid, 17
Transverse lie, 110, 112
Trimester, assessment of, 26, 27, 28

# U

Ultrasound, 10, 31, 73
umbilical cord, 8, 128
    prolapsed, 129
Universal Precautions, 195
Urinary Tract Infection, 15, 55, 64, 65, 163
Urination, 51, 55
uterine contraction, 119
Uterine inversion, 110
Uterine involution, 152
Uterine position, 11, 137
Uterine rupture, 108, 109
Uterine shape, 137
Uterine tone, 11, 137
Uterus, 11, 13, 136, 147
    uterine atony, 157
    Uterine involution, 152
    Uterine inversion, 161
    Uterine position, 137
    Uterine shape, 137
    Uterine tone, 137

# V

Vagina, 12, 138
Vaginal infection, 56
Variable Decelerations, 42
Varicose veins, 53
vena cava syndrome, 13
Vernix Caseosa, 9, 180, 204
Vital statistics, 186
Vital signs, 146, 185
Vitamin K synthesis, 177, 195
Vitamins, 61
Vomiting, 14, 51, 64, 74

# W

Weight
       Low birth, 191
Weight gain, 29, 57, 92
White's classification, 61, 70

# Z

zygote, 6

|  | CODE | ISBN # | PRICE | QTY |
|---|---|---|---|---|
| **INSTANT INSTRUCTOR SERIES** | | | | |
| AIDS/HIV | ADIN01 | 1-56930-010-0 | $16.95 | |
| C.C.U. | CCINC1 | 1-56930-022-4 | 16.95 | |
| Diabetes | DBII01 | 1-56930-041-0 | 16.95 | |
| Geriatric | GRN01 | 0-944132-68-5 | 16.95 | |
| Hemodialysis | DLIN01 | 1-56930-020-8 | 16.95 | |
| I.C.U. | ICUI01 | 1-56930-021-6 | 16.95 | |
| IV | IVII01 | 1-56930-043-7 | 16.95 | |
| Lab | LBIN01 | 0-944132-70-7 | 16.95 | |
| Obstetric | OBIN01 | 0-944132-67-7 | 16.95 | |
| Oncology | ONIN01 | 1-56930-023-2 | 16.95 | |
| Pediatric | PDIN01 | 0-944132-66-9 | 16.95 | |
| **NURSE'S SURVIVAL GUIDE SERIES** | | | | |
| Nurse's Survival Guide (2nd ed.) | NSGD02 | 0-944132-75-8 | 32.95 | |
| Geriatric Nurses' Survival Guide | GSGD01 | 1-56930-061-5 | 29.95 | |
| Obstetric Survival Guide | OBSG01 | 0-944132-94-4 | 29.95 | |
| Pediatric Survival Guide | PNGD01 | 1-56930-018-6 | 29.95 | |
| **OUTLINE SERIES** | | | | |
| Diabetes Outline | DBOL01 | 1-56930-031-3 | 22.95 | |
| Fundamentals of Nursing Outline | FUND01 | 1-56930-029-1 | 22.95 | |
| Geriatric Outline | GER01 | 1-56930-050-x | 22.95 | |
| Hemodynamic Monitoring Outline | HDMO01 | 1-56930-034-8 | 22.95 | |
| High Acuity Outline | HATO01 | 1-56930-028-3 | 22.95 | |
| Medical-Surgical Nursing Outline (2nd ed.) | MSN02 | 1-56930-068-2 | 22.95 | |
| Obstetric Nursing Outline (2nd ed.) | OBS02 | 1-56930-070-4 | 22.95 | |
| Pediatric Nursing Outline | PN01 | 0-944132-89-8 | 22.95 | |
| **NURSING CARE PLANS SERIES** | | | | |
| AIDS/HIV | ADSC01 | 1-56930-000-3 | 36.95 | |
| Critical Care | CNCP01 | 1-56930-035-6 | 36.95 | |
| Geriatric (2nd ed.) | GNCP02 | 1-56930-052-6 | 36.95 | |
| Oncology | ONCP01 | 1-56930-004-6 | 36.95 | |
| Pediatric (2nd ed.) | PNOP02 | 1-56930-057-7 | 36.95 | |

|  | CODE | ISBN # | PRICE | QTY |
|---|---|---|---|---|
| **RN NCLEX REVIEW SERIES** | | | | |
| Concepts of Medical Surgical Nursing | NMS01 | 0-944132-85-5 | 21.95 | |
| Concepts of Obstetric Nursing | NOB01 | 0-944132-86-3 | 21.95 | |
| Concepts of Psychiatric Nursing | NPSY01 | 0-944132-83-9 | 21.95 | |
| PN/VN Review Cards (2nd ed.) | PNRC02 | 1-56930-008-9 | 29.95 | |
| RN Review Cards (2nd ed.) | RNRC02 | 0-944132-82-0 | 29.95 | |
| **NURSING/OTHER** | | | | |
| Body In Brief (3rd ed.) | BBRF03 | 1-56930-055-0 | 35.95 | |
| Diagnostic and Lab Cards (2nd ed.) | DLC02 | 0-944132-77-4 | 27.95 | |
| Drug Comparison Handbook (2nd ed.) | DRUG02 | 1-56930-16-x | 35.95 | |
| Essential Laboratory Mathematics | ELM01 | 1-56930-056-9 | 29.95 | |
| Geriatric Long-Term Procedures & Treatments | GLTP01 | 0-944132-97-9 | 34.95 | |
| Geriatric Nutrition and Diet (2nd ed.) | NUT02 | 1-56930-045-3 | 17.95 | |
| Handbook of Long-Term Care (2nd ed.) | HLTC02 | 1-56930-058-5 | 22.95 | |
| Handbook for Nurse Assistants (2nd ed.) | HNA02 | 1-56930-059-3 | 19.95 | |
| I.C.U. Quick Reference | ICQU01 | 1-56930-003-8 | 32.95 | |
| Infection Control | INFC01 | 1-56930-051-8 | 94.95 | |
| Nursing Diagnosis Cards (2nd ed.) | NDC02 | 1-56930-060-7 | 29.95 | |
| Nurse's Trivia Calendar 1998 | NTC98 | 1-56930-073-9 | 11.95 | |
| OBRA (2nd ed.) | OBRA02 | 1-56930-046-1 | 99.95 | |
| OSHA Book (2nd ed.) | OSHA02 | 1-56930-069-0 | 119.95 | |
| Procedure Cards (3rd ed.) | PCCU03 | 1-56930-054-2 | 24.95 | |
| Pharmacy Tech | PHAR01 | 1-56930-005-4 | 25.95 | |
| Spanish for Medical Personnel | SPAN01 | 1-56930-001-1 | 21.95 | |
| Staff Development for the Psychiatric Nurse | STDEV01 | 0-944132-78-2 | 59.95 | |
| (prices subject to change at any given time) | | | | |

| | | |
|---|---|---|
| Amount of Order | $ | _____ |
| Shipping & Handling | | $6.95 |
| Local Sales Tax | $ | _____ |
| | | |
| Order Total | $ | _____ |

# ORDER FORM

Name _____

Address _____

City _____ State ____ Zip _____

Phone (        ) _____

☐ Visa ☐ Mastercard ☐ American Express ☐ Check/Money Order

Card Number _____

Expiration Date _____

Signature _____

Please add $6.95 for shipping and handling.
Please include your local sales tax.
Prices subject to change at any time.

**Skidmore-Roth Publishing, Inc.**
2620 S. Parker Road, Suite 147
Aurora, Colorado 80014
Toll free: 1-800-825-3150
Fax: 303-306-1460

Visit our website at: http//www.skidmore-roth.com